BODY Acupuncture

CLINICAL TREATMENT

针炎临床治疗

Sumiko Knudsen

Ph.D
Practitioner.DK

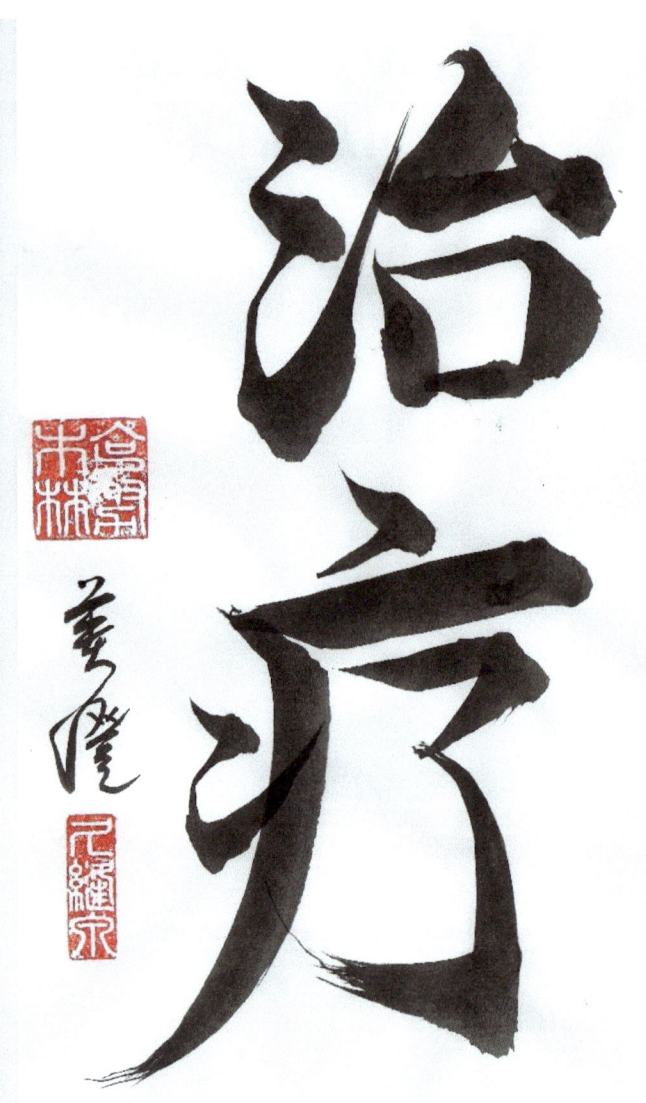

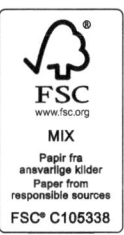

© 2021 Knudsen, Sumiko
Forlag: BoD – Books on Demand, København, Danmark
Tryk: BoD – Books on Demand, Norderstedt, Tyskland

ISBN: 9788743030430

CONTENTS

6

10

INTRODUCTION

In Therapeutics of acupuncture, acupuncture points are the places where acupuncture needle is applied for the treatment of diseases. This acupuncture point location and the therapeutic result are related.

The processing is done by inserting thin disposable needles into specific points relating to the internal organs. In this way body is activated with flow of Qi (energy).

This book guides by the principles governing the prescription and combination of points of Acupuncture, and it lets to find easily acupuncture points of diseases. It introduces more than 100 common diseases, and it is handy to use.

The locations of acupuncture points are certainly related to physiological functions. Stimulating acupoints in meridians of the affected area may be effective and stimulate meridian points for each disease to approach the affected area. Stimulation through acupuncture points can correct imbalance and blockages in the flow of energy for restoring health.

Sumiko Knudsen 克努森澄子

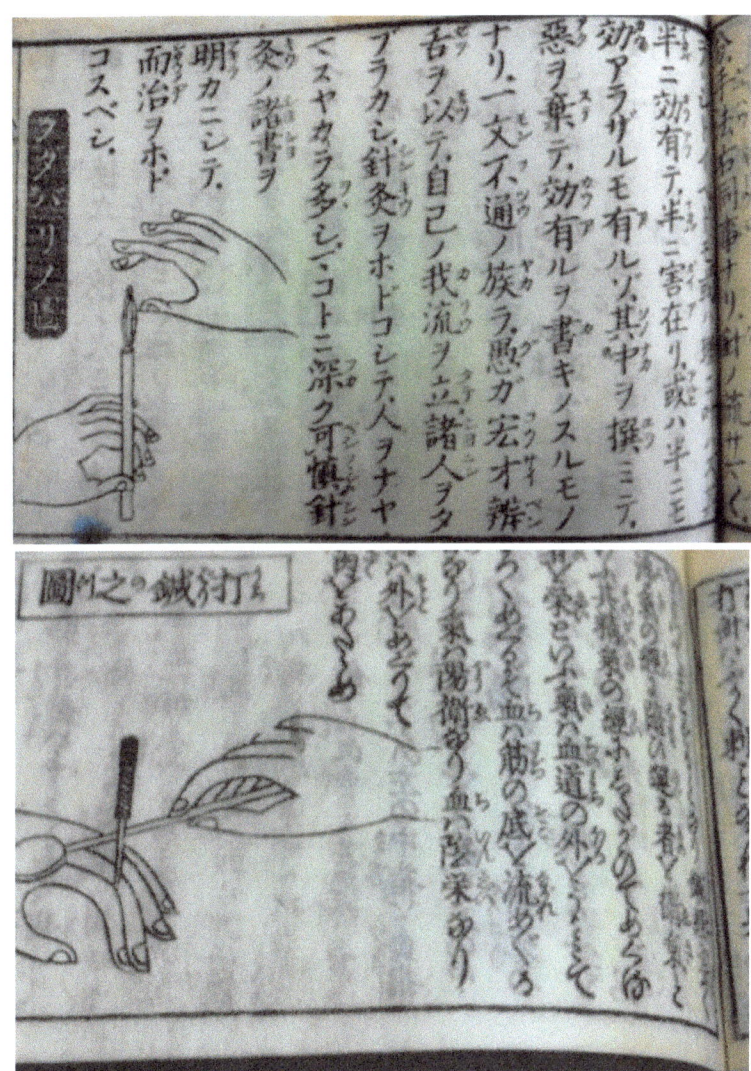

半ニ効有テ半ニ害在リ或ハ半ニモ
効アラザルモ有ルゾ其中ヲ撰ニテ
悪ヲ棄テ効有ルヲ書キノスルモノ
ナリ一文不通ノ族ラ悪ガ宏才辨
舌ヲ以テ自己ノ我流ヲ立諸人ヲタ
ブラカシ針灸ヲホドコシテ人ヲナヤ
マスヤカラ多シテコトニ深ク可愼針
灸ノ諸書ヲ
明カニシテ
而治ヲホド
コスベシ。

フタゝペ刀之圖

圖州之の鍼打る

Edo period about 1600

- In alphabetic order -

Charpter 1   Internal Medicine

1-1 Abdominal Pain 腹痛 Futong

- **Differentiation**

1. Internal accumulation of cold:
   Sudden violent pain which responds to warmth and is aggravated by cold. Other manifestations include loose stools, profuse clear urine, white coated tongue, deep tense or deep slow pulse.

2. Retention of food:
   Epigastric and abdominal distension and pain which may be aggravated by pressure, foul belching and acidity. Abdominal pain may be accompanied by diarrhea and relieved after defecation. The tongue is sticky coated, the pulse is rolling.

- **Treatment**

   Prescriptions
1. Accumulation of Cold in the interior

REN-12 (Zhongwan 中脘), REN-8 (Shenque 神闕)，ST-36 (Zusanli 足三里)

2. Retention of food
Prescription:

REN-10 (Xianwan 下脘), ST-21 (Liangmen 梁門), (Gongsun 公孫), ST-36 (Zusanli 足三里)

3. Deficiency of Spleen Yang

Prescription:

BL-20 (Pishu 脾俞), BL-21 (Weishu 胃俞), REN-12 (Zhongwan 中脘), REN-4 （Guanyuan 关元）, REN-6 (Qihai 气海), LIV-13 (Zhangmen 章门)

- **Addition**

Pain above the umbilicus:
REN-10 (Xiawan 下脘), ST-36 (Zusanli 足三里)

Pain around the umbilicus:
ST-25 (Tianshu 天枢), REN-6 (Qihai 气海)

Pain in the lower abdomen:

REN-4 (Guanyuan 关元), SP-6(Sanyinjiao 三阴交)

- **Remarks**

By acute and severe abdominal pain, it is necessary to have the strict observation of the patient, and other therapeutic measures should be taken.

- **Ear acupuncture**

Large Intestine, Small Intestine, Shenmen, Subcortex, Spleen

1-2 Abdominal Distension 腹胀 Fuzhang

- **Differentiation**

1. Excess Type:
The persistent distention and fullness in the abdomen, which may also cause abdominal pain, is aggravated by pressing. It is accompanied by belching, foul breathing, dark

yellow urine, constipation or occasional fever and vomiting, yellow thick tongue coating, and slippery rapid and forceful pulse.

2. Deficiency Type:
It is accompanied by borborygmus, loose stool, poor appetite, general lassitude, poor sprit, clear urine, pale tongue proper with white coating and feeble pulse.

- **Treatment**

1. Excess Type:

Prescription:

REN-12 (Zhongwan 中脘), ST-25 (Tianshu 天樞), ST-36 (Zusanli 足三里), ST-37 (Shangjuxu 上巨虚)

2. Deficiency Type:

Prescription:

REN-11 (Jianli 建里), REN-4 (Guanyuan 关元), ST-25 (Tianshu 天枢), ST-36 (Zusanli 足三里), SP-3 (Taibai 太白)

- **Remarks**

  Abdominal distention is mostly caused by impairment of the Spleen and Stomach due to irregular or excessive food intake, resulting in dysfunction of transportation and transformation. The food retention forms and obstructs the Qi mechanism, giving rise to a distending sensation in the abdomen.

- **Ear acupuncture**

  Spleen, Stomach, Large Intestine, Small Intestine, Sympathetic, Subcortex

1-3 Angina Pectoris 心绞痛 Xinjiaotong

- **Differentiation**

1. Angina Pectoris is the main syndrome of coronary atherosclerotic cardiopathy. The main clinical manifestations include paroxysmal pain or oppressed feeling in the precordial area, radiating to the left shoulder, left arm, or to the neck and throat. It is

induced by physical exertion, emotional disturbance, over-eating or attach by cold, and relieved by rest and treatment.

- **Treatment**

  Prescription:
  P-6 (Neiguan 内关), P-4 (Ximen 郄门), Ren-17 (Danzhong 膻中), ST-36 (Zusanli 足三里), BL-44 (Shentang 神堂)

1-4 Asthma 哮喘 Xiaochuan

- **Differentiation**

1. Wind-Cold in the Lung:
   The main manifestations include difficult respiration, cough with shortness of breath and wheezing sound in the throat, dilute sputum of white colour, cold limbs without sweating, greyish facial complexion, white or white greasy tongue coating, and superficial

tense or superficial slippery pulse. It may be accompanied by chills, fever, headache.

2. Phlegm-Heat Retention in the Lung:
The main manifestations include shallow breathing, strong and coarse voice, cough with thick yellow sputum, stuffy sensation in the chest and epigastric region. It is accompanied by fever, dryness of the mouth, thirst with desire for cold drinking, yellow greasy or sticky coating tongue and rapid slippery pulse.

- **Treatment**

1. Wind-Cold in the lung:

Prescription:

LU-7 (Lieque 列缺), BL-13 (Feishu 肺俞), BL-12 (Fengmen 风门), ST-9 (Renying 人迎), EX-B1 (Dingchuan 定喘)

2. Phlegm-Heat Retention in the Lung:

Prescription:

LU-5 (Chize 尺泽), LU-6 (Kongzui 孔最), DU-14 (Dazhui 大椎), ST-40 (Fenglong 丰隆), LI-4 (Hegu 合谷), REN-17 (Danzhong 膻中)

- **Remarks**

This condition includes bronchial asthma, asthmatic bronchitis, obstructive pulmonary emphysema and dyspnea. For severe dyspnea, it is necessary to have a combined treatment.

- **Ear acupuncture**

Lung, Trachea, Subcortex Sympathetic, Adrenal gland, Shenmen, Endcrine

- **Empirical acupuncture points**

DU-20 (Baihui 百会), DU-14 (Dazhui 大椎), REN-17 (Shanzhong 膻中), Ren-19 (Zigong 子宫), LU-1 (Zhongfu 中风), LU-2 (Yunmen 云门), Ren-9 (Shuifen 水分), ST-25 (Tianshu 天枢), LU-5 (Chize 尺泽), LU-7 (Lieque 列缺), SP-10 (Xuehai 血海), SP-9 (Yinlingquan 阴陵泉), KI-3

(Taixi 太溪), ST-41 (Jiexi 解溪), LIV-3 (Taichong 太冲), ST-40 (Fenglong 丰隆)

1-5 Aphonia 失音 Shiyin

- **Differentiation**

1. Excess Type

(1) Wind-Cold:
   The sudden hoarseness of voice is accompanied by difficult cough, fullness in the chest, stuffy nose, chills, fever, headache, with thin white tongue coating and superficial pulse.

(2) Phlegm-Heat:
   The sudden low voice or husky voice is accompanied by cough, yellow sputum, sore throat, dry nose, fever, thirst, thin yellow tongue coating and rapid superficial pulse.

(3) Qi Stagnation:

The sudden aphonia that is often induced by emotional upset such as sorrow, grief, depression or anger appears paroxysmal. It is accompanied by restlessness, irritability, suffocating sensation in the chest, or a foreign body sensation in the throat, thin yellow tongue coating and thready pulse.

2. Deficient Type
The progressive aphonia is accompanied by dry throat, thirst, tidal fever, night sweating, dry cough, palpitation, dizziness, tinnitus, red tongue with less coating, and thin rapid pulse.

- **Treatment**

1. Excess Type

(1) Wind-Cold:
LU-7 (Lieque 列缺), LI-4 (Hegu 合谷), LI-17 (Tianding 天鼎), ST-9 (Renying 人迎)

(2) Phlegm-Heat:
LU-10 (Yuji 鱼际), ST-40 (Fenglong 豐隆), ST-9 (Renying 人迎), LI-17 (Tianding 天鼎), REN-22 (Tiantu 天突)

(3) Qi Stagnation:

LIV-3 (Taichong 太冲), SJ-6 (Zhigou 支沟), SJ-1 (Guanchong 关冲), ST-9 (Renying 人迎)

2. Deficient Type

LU-10 (Yuji 鱼际), LU-7 (Lieque 列缺), ST-9 (Renying 人迎), KI-6 (Zhaohai 照海), KI-3 (Taixi 太溪)

- **Remarks**

The patient should take light taste food, and all kinds of spicy and fried food should be avoided, such as pepper, garlic, spring onion and fried food.

- **Ear acupuncture**

Lung, Kidney, Throat Trochea, Large Intestine

1-6 Appendicitis 阑尾炎 Lanweiyan

- **Manifestation**

  There is mainly pain at the center of the umbilicus or around the umbilicus in the right lower abdomen. It is accompanied by fever, nausea diarrhea, vomiting, distension, rapid pulse.

- **Treatment**

  Prescription
  Ashi point (阿是)
  ST-25 (Tianshu 天枢), ST-37 (Shangjuxu 上巨虚), EX-LE6 (Lanwei 阑尾)

  Fever:
  LI-4 (Hegu 合谷), LI-11 (Quchi 曲池)
  Vomitting:
  ST-44 (Neiting 内庭), REN-12 (Zhongwan 中脘)

  Abdominal Distension:
  SP-15 (Daheng 大横), REN-6 (Qihai 气海)

- **Remarks**

  It refers to Intestinal Abscess (Changyong 肠痈).

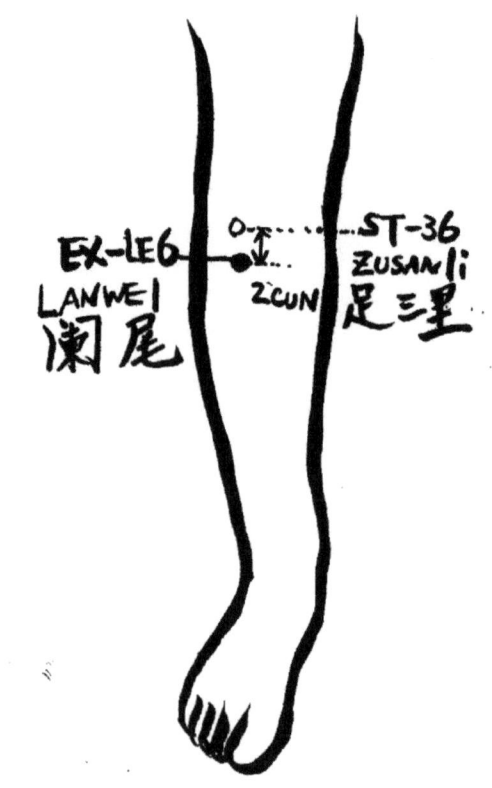

1-7 BI Syndrome 痹症 Bizheng

- **Differentiation**

  The main symptom is arthralgia, including soreness and numbness in the body limbs, joints and muscles, particularly in the wrist joints, elbow, knee and ankle areas. In prolonged cases, contracture of the extremities, or even swelling or deformity of joints may occur.

- **Treatment**

  Prescriptin: Based on diseased/pain area.
  Shoulder:
  LI-15 (Jianyu 肩髃), SJ14 (Jianliao 肩髎), SI-10 (Naoshu 臑俞), LI-4 (Hegu 合谷)

  Elbow:
  LI-11 (Quchi 曲池), SJ-10 (Tianjing 天井), LU-5 (Chize 尺泽), SJ-5 (Waiguan 外关)

  Wrist:
  LI-5 (Yangxi 阳溪), SJ-4 (Yangchi 阳池), SJ-5 (Waiguan 外关), SI-4 (Wangu 腕骨)

Hip:
GB-30 (Huantiao 环跳), GB-29 (Juliao 居髎),
GB-39 (Xuanzhong 悬钟)

Knee:
ST-34 (Liangqiu 梁丘), SP-10 (Xuehai 血海), SP-9 (Yinlingquan 阴陵泉), GB-34 (Yanglingquan 阳陵泉), EX-LE4 (Xiyan 膝眼)

Ankle:
ST-41 (Jiexi 解溪), SP-5 (Shangqiu 商丘), BL-60 (Kunlun 昆仑), KI-3 (Taixi 太溪), GB-40 (Qiuxu 丘墟)
Lumbar region:
DU-3 (Yaoyangguan 腰阳关), DU-12 (Shenzhu 身柱), DU-14 (Dazhui 大椎), EX-B1 (jiaji 夹脊)

- **Remarks**

BI syndrome may be seen in rheumatic fever, rheumatic arthritis, and rheumatoid arthritis.

- **Moxibution**

REN-8 (Shenque 神阙) with ginger slice with small holes may apply.

1-8 Beriberi 脚气 Jiaoqi

- **Differentiation**

1. Damp type

   The main manifestations include swelling of foot dorsum, pain and numbness of toes which gradually affects the legs. It is difficulty in walking with soreness, heaviness with knee joints and weakness of the feet. There will be feverish sensation in dorsum of the feet that responds to cooling if the damp-heat is more prevailing. The damp-heat type may include fever with aversion to cold, short scanty urine, white greasy or slightly yellow tongue coating, rapid pulse.

2. Dry type

   The main manifestations include weakness of both feet, numbness and pain of legs and knees with occasional tendon spasm, limited movement, gradual atrophy of foot muscles, constipation, yellow urinary discharge, slightly red tongue, thin white tongue coating, and rapid thready pulse.

3. Affecting the Heart

The main manifestations include swelling, pain or numbness with atrophy and weakness for walking, sudden onset of shortness of breath, palpitation, nausea, vomiting, restlessness, purplish lips, rapid thready pulse.

- **Treatment**

Prescription
1. Damp type
   ST-36 (Zusanli 足三里), SP-6 (Sanyinjiao 三阴交), GB-34 (Yanglingquan 阳陵泉), EX-LE10 (Bafeng 八风)

2. Dry type
   ST-41 (Jiexi 解溪), ST-33 (Yinshi 阴市), KI-7 (Fuliu 复瘤), KI-6 (Zaohai 照海), SP-10 (Xuehai 血海), GB-39 (Xuanzhong 悬钟)

3. Affecting the Heart
   LU-5 (Chize 尺泽), REN-17 (Danzhong 膻中), P-8 (Laogong 劳宫), HT-7 (Shenmen 神门), ST-36 (Zusanli 足三里), KI-1 (Yongquan 涌泉)

- **Remarks**

  Beriberi refers to flaccid, swollen feet and lower portion of the legs, or weakness and numbness of the feet. It can be referred to that feet malnutrition and polyneuritis are similar manifestations.

- **Ear acupuncture**

  Stomach, Spleen, Shenmen, Kidney, Lung, Ankle, Knee, Toe

1-9 Back Pain 背痛 Beitong

- **Differentiation**

  The exogenous factor mainly refers to the pathogenic wind-cold invading, causing blockage in the meridians, Qi and Blood circulation, and becomes back pain.

- **Treatment**

Prescription:
DU-14 (Dazhui 大椎), DU-12 (Shenzhu 身柱), Du-9 (Zhiyang 至阳), Extra (Jiaji 夹脊), Ashi point, BL-40 (Weizhong 委中), BL-60 (Kunlun 昆仑)

- **Remarks**
  It is seen in the spondylitis in modern medicine.

1-10 Biliary Disorders (Acute)

- **Manifestation**

  It is colic pain in the right upper abdomen which radiate to the right shoulder, and also upper back, accompanied by nausea, vomiting, fever and jaundice.

- **Treatment**

  ST-36 (Zusanli 足三里), GB-34 (Yanglingquan 阳陵泉), GB-40 (Qiuxu 丘墟), BL-18 (Ganshu 肝

俞), BL-19 (Danshu 胆俞), EX-LE6 (Dannang 胆
囊)

- **Remarks**

Acute Biliary Disorders belong to
Hypochondriac (Xietong 胁痛) pain and
Jaudice (Huangdan 黄胆).

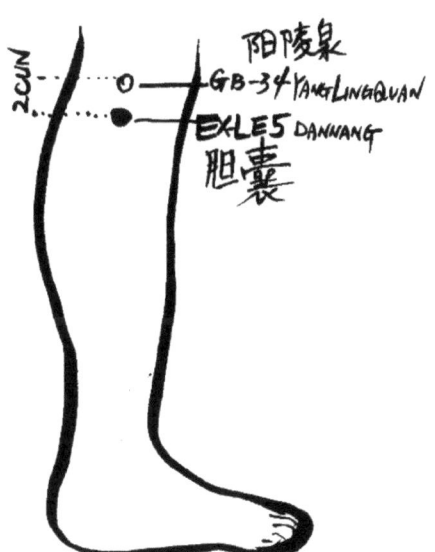

1-11 Chest Bi Syndrom 胸痹 Xiongbizheng

- **Differentiation**

1. Deficient Cold Type
   The main manifestations include chest pain aggravated by cold and radiating towards the back, palpitation, fullness sensation in the chest, shortness of breath, aversion to cold, white greasy tongue coating, deep thin pulse.

2. Turbid Phlegm Retention Type
   The main manifestations include stuffy sensation, chest pain towards the back and shoulder, fullness in the epigastrium and abdomen, listlessness, palpitation, shortness of breath, cough, profuse white sticky sputum, white greasy tongue coating, soft slow pulse.

3. Blood Stasis Type
   The main manifestations include pricking pain in the chest radiating towards the shoulder and back, fullness of the chest, shortness of breath, palpitation, dark tongue, thin uneven pulse.

- **Treatment**

Prescription
1. Deficient Cold Type
   BL-15 (Xinshu 心俞), REN-14 (Juque 巨阙), BL-14 (Jueyinshu 厥阴俞), REN-17 (Danzhong 膻中), P-6 (Neiguan 内关), HT-5 (Tongli 通里)

2. Turbid Phlegm
   REN-14 (Juque 巨阙), REN-17 (Danzhong 膻中), P-4 (Ximen 郄门), REN-11 (Jianli 建里), ST-40 (Fenglong 豐隆), SP-5 (Sanyinjiao 三阴交)

3. Blood Stasis Type
   DU-9 (Zhiyang 至阳), HT-6 (Yinxi 阴郄), BL-15 (Xinshu 心俞), REN-14 (Juque 巨阙), BL-17 (Geshu 膈俞), REN-17 (Danzhong 膻中)

- **Remarks**

It is closely related to the dysfunction of heart and lungs as anatomical way. It is commonly seen in coronary arteriosclerotic cardiopathy in modern medicine.

- **Ear acupuncture**

  Heart, Small Intestine, Sympathetic, Subcortex, Lung, Chest, Shenmen

1-12 Common Cold 普通感 Putongganmao

- **Differentiation**

1. Wind-Cold Type
   Mild fever without sweating, aversion to cold, headache, running nose, cough, thin whitish Sputum, thin white tongue coating, rapid superficial pulse.

2. Wind-Heat Type
   High fever, spontaneous sweating, headache, stuffy nose, sore throat, dry mouth with desire for drinking, cough with yellowish thick sputum, thin yellow tongue coating, rapid superficial pulse.

3. Damp-Heat Type

The Main manifestations are high fever without sweating, headache, fullness sensation in the chest, lassitude, nausea, anorexia, abdominal distention, loose stool, sticky whitish sputum, thick yellow tongue coating, soft rapid pulse.

- **Treatment**

Prescription
1. Wind-Cold Type
   LU-7 (Lieque 列缺), BL-12 (fengmen 风门), GB-20 (Fengchi 凤池), LI-4 (Hegu 合谷)
2. Wind-Heat Type
   LU-5 (Chize 尺泽), LU-10 (Yuji 鱼际), LI-4 (Hegu 合谷), LI-11 (Quchi 曲池), DU-14 Dazhui 大椎)

3. Damp-Heat type
   LU-6 (Kongzui 孔最), LI-4 (Hegu 合谷), REN-12 (Zhongwan 中脘), ST-36 (Zusanli 足三里), SJ-5 (Waiguan 外关)

- **Remarks**

It may occur around the year, and this condition includes bacterial infection in modern medicine.

Ear acupuncture:
Lung, Throat, Ear apex, Trachea, Internal nose, Stomach, Sanjiao, Spleen, Adrenal gland, Subcortex

1-13 Cough 咳嗽 Kesou

• **Differentiation**

1. Exopathogenic Factors
(1) Wind-Cold Type
It is characterized by itching sensation in the throat. It is accompanied by fever, chills, headache, nasal obstruction, soreness of joints. The tongue has thin white coating, and superficial pulse.

(2) Wind-Heat Type
Fever without chills, thirst, cough with thick sputum, dry mouth and sticky yellowish

sputum, tongue with yellowish coating, rapid superficial pulse.

2. Endopathogenic Factors
(1) Yang Deficiency with Spleen
Cough with excessive sputum, fullness sensation in the chest and epigastric region, listlessness, white greasy tongue coating, deep and slow pulse.

(1) Yin Deficiency with Dryness of the Lung
Dry cough without sputum, dry throat, feverish palms and soles, fever, red tongue with thin coating, feeble rapid pulse.

- **Treatment**

Prescription:
1. Exopathogenic Factors
(1) Wind-Cold Type
LU-7 (Lieque 列缺), LI-4 (Hegu 合谷), BL-13 (Feishu 肺俞), SJ-5 (Waiguan 外关)
(2) Wind-Heat Type
LU-5 (Chize 尺泽), LI-11 (Quchi 曲池), DU-14 (Dazhui 大椎), BL-13 (Feishu 肺俞)

2. Endopathogenic Factors

(1) Yang Deficiency with Spleen

LU-9 (Taiyuan 太渊), SP-3 (Taibai 太白), ST-40 (Fenglong 丰隆), BL-13 (Feishu 肺俞), BL-20 (Pishu 脾俞)

(2) Yin Deficiency with Dryness of the Lung

LU-1 (Zhongfu 中府), LU-7 (Lieque 列缺), BL-13 (Feishu 肺俞), KI-6 (Zhaohai 照海), LIV-3 (Taichong 太冲)

- **Remarks**

  It is a symptom indicating the impaired function of the Lung which descending and dispersing.

- **Ear acupuncture**

  Lung, Bonchea, Occipit, Spleen, Kidney, Sympathetic, Adrenal gland, Shenmen

- **Empirical points**

  DU-20 (Baihui 百会), DU-23 (Shangxing 上星), REN-19 (Zigong 子宫), LU-1 (Zhongfu 中府), SJ-

5 (Waiguan 外关), LI-11 (Quchi 曲池), ST-36 (Zusanli 足三里), LIV-3 (Taichoong 太冲), KI-7 (Fuliu 复瘤), ST-38 (Tiaokou 条口)

1-14 Constipation 便秘 Bianmi

- **Differentiation**

1. Heat Type
   Absence of bowel motions for several days, abdominal pain, fullness and distention, restlessness, dry mouth with foul breath, yellow tong coating, rapid slippery pulse.

2. Qi Stagnation Type
   Frequent bowel movements, distending pain in the abdomen, bitter taste, dizziness, poor appetite, thin greasy tongue coating, thready pulse.

3. Deficient Type
   Dry stool difficult to discharge, shortness of breath and lassitude, no distention and pain

of abdomen, palpitation, dizziness, blurred vision, pale tongue, thin coating, thin feeble pulse.

4. Cold Type
   Dry stool difficult to discharge, occasional pain of abdomen, cold limbs, clear urine, pale tongue with white coating, deep slow pulse.

- **Treatment**

Prescription
1. Heat Type
   LI-4 (Hegu 合谷), LI-11 (Quchi 曲池), ST-25 tianshu 天枢), ST-44 (Neiting 内庭), SP-14 (Fujie 腹結)
   ST-37 (Shangjuxu)

2. Qi Stagnation Type
   REN-12 (Zhongwan 中脘), ST-25 (Tianshu 天枢), GB-34 (Yanglingquan 阳陵泉), SJ-6 (Zhigou 支沟), LIV-2 (Xingjian 行间)

3. Deficient Type
   REN-4 (Guanyuan 关元), REN-6 (Qihai 气海), BL-20 (Pishu 脾俞), BL-21 (Weishu 胃俞), ST-36 (Zusanli 足三里)

4. Cold Type Prescription
   REN-6 (Qihai 气海), REN-8 (Shenque 神阙), ST-25 (Tianshu 天枢), KI-6 (Zhaohai 照海), BL-23 (Shenshu 肾俞)

- **Ear acupuncture**

  Lung, Spleen, Large Intestine, Subcortex, Rectum, Constipation point

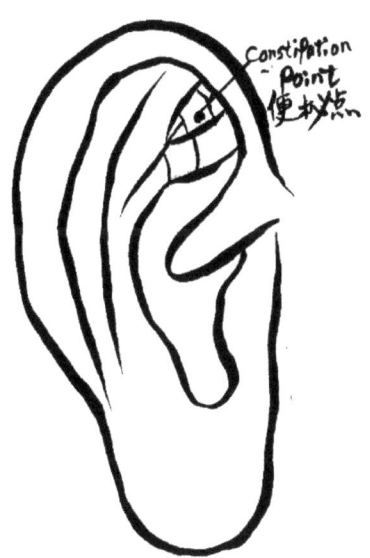

1-15 Diarrhea 泄泻 Xiexie

- **Differenciation**

1. Acute Diarrhea

(1) Cold-Damp Type
Loose stools with abdominal pain, borborygmus, cold with desire for warmth, absence of thirst, pale tongue with white coating, deep and slow pulse.

(2) Damp-Heat Type
Loose stools with abdominal pain, urgent bowel motion, feverish sensation in the anus, scanty urine, yellow greasy tongue coating, rapid slippery soft pulse.

2. Chronic Diarrhea

(1) Spleen Yang Deficiency
Loose stools with undigested food, abdominal and epigastric distension, anorexia, lassitude, white sticky tongue coating, soft slow pulse.

(2) Kidney Yang Deficiency

Abdominal pain, borborygmus and diarrhea before dawn, cold extremities, white tongue coating, deep forceless pulse.

- **Treatment**

Prescription
1. Acute Diarrhea
(1) Cold-Damp type
ST-25 (Tianshu 天枢), ST-37 (Shangjuxu 上巨虚), REN-6 (Qihai 气海), REN-11 (Jianli 建里), SP-9 (Yinlingquan 阴陵泉)

(2) Damp-Heat Type
ST-44 (Neiting 内庭), ST-25 (Tianshu 天枢), REN-12 (Zhongwan 中脘), SP-9 (Yinlingquan 阴陵泉), LI-11 (Quchi 曲池)

2. Chronic Diarrhea
(1) Spleen Yang Deficiency
SP-3 (Taibai 太白), ST-25 (Tianshu 天枢), ST-36 (Zusanli 足三里), BL-20 (Pishu 脾俞), REN-12 (Zhongwan 中脘), LIV-13 (Zhangmen 章门)

(2) Kidney Yang Deficiency

BL-20 (Pishu 脾俞), BL-23 (Shenshu 肾俞), DU-4 (Mingmen 命门), REN-4 (Guanyuan 关元), ST-25 (Tianshu 天枢), ST-37 (Shangjuxu 上巨虚)

- **Remarks**

It is mainly caused by dysfunctions of the Spleen and Stomach.

Ear Acupuncture:
Large Intestine, Small Intestine, Stomach, Spleen Liver, Kidney, Sympathetic, Shenmen

1-16 Dizziness 眩晕 Xuanyun

- **Differentiation**
1. Hyperactivity of Liver Yang
   The manifestations are tinnitus, nausea, backache disturbed sleep, flushed face, congested eyes, red tongue proper with thin yellow coating, wiry rapid pulse.

2. Qi and Blood Deficiency

The manifestations are palpitation, insomnia, pale complexion, pale complexion, poor appetite, pale tongue proper, weak pulse.

3. Phlegm-Damp obstruction in the interior
The manifestations are lassitude, fullness in the chest and epigastrium, heaviness of head, vomiting, white and sticky tongue, rolling pulse.

- **Treatment**

Prescription

1. Hyperactivity of Liver Yang
GB-20 (Fengchi 凤池), GB-43 (Xiaxi 侠溪), LIV-3 (Taichong 太冲), BL-18 (Ganshu 肝俞)

2. Qi and Blood Deficiency
BL-20 (Pishu 脾俞), BL-23 (Shenshu 肾俞), ST-36 (Zusanli 足三里), SP-6 (Sanyinjiao 三阴交), REN-4 (Guanyuan 关元), DU-20 (Baihui 百会)

3. Phlegm-Damp obstruction in the interior
REN-12 (Zhongwan 中脘), DU-20 (Baihui 百会), BL-20 (Pishu 脾俞), P-6 (Neiguan 内关), ST-36 (Zusanli 足三里), ST-40 (Fenglong 丰隆)

- **Remarks**

  It can be seen in hypertension, anemia, neurasthenia, arteriosclerosis etc.

- **Ear acupuncture**
  Kidney, Shenmen, Subcortex, Inner ear

1-17 Dysentery 痢疾 Liji

- **Differentiation**

1. Damp-Heat Type
   The manifestations are abdominal pain,white and red mucus in stool, burning sensation in the anus, high fever in severe case. Tongue is mostly yellow and sticky coated, rapid rolling pulse.
2. Cold-Damp Type
   The manifestations are fullness in the chest and epigastrium, tastelessness, absence of thirst, white and red mucus in stool, white greasy tongue coating, rapid deep slow pulse.

3. Chronic Dysentery
   This is a kind of recurrent dysentery. There may be lassitude, cold limbs, sallow complexion, greasy tongue coating, deep thready pulse.

- **Treatment**

  Prescription
  1. Damp-Heat Type
     ST-25 (Tianshu 天枢), ST-37 (Shangjuxu 上巨虚), ST-44 (Neiting 内庭), Li-4 (Hegu 合谷)

  2. Cold-Damp Type
     SP-9 (Yinlingquan 阴陵泉), ST-25 (Tianshu 天枢), ST-37 (Shangjuxu 上巨虚), REN-6 (Qihai 气海), REN-12 (Zhongwan 中脘)

  3. Chronic Dysentery
     ST-25 (Tianshu 天枢), ST-36 (Zusanli 足三里), BL-20 (Pishu 脾俞), BL-21 (Weishu 胃俞), BL-25 (Dachangshu 大肠俞), REN-4 (Guanyuan 关元)

- **Remarks**

It is an intestinal epidemic disease which causes in the summer. It is characterized by abdominal pain. Bowel motion contains often blood and mucous.

- **Ear acupuncture**
  Kidney, Spleen, Stomach, Large Intestine, Small Intestine, Rectum

1-18 Depressive Manic Mental Disorders
抑郁性燥狂症 **Yiyuxingzaokuangzheng**

- **Differentiation**

(1) Depressive mental disorders
Gradual onset, mental depression and dullness at the initial stage. It is followed by paraphasia, muteness, hypersomnia and anorexia, illusions. Tongue is thin greasy coating, and thready and wiry pulse.

(2) Manic mental disorders
Sudden onset proceeds by irritability, less sleep and no desire for eating. The

manifestation followed by shouting, violent behavior, destroying the objects and harming people. Yellow greasy tongue coating, and rapid slippery pulse.

- **Treatment**

Prescription
(1) Depressive mental disorders
BL-15 (Xinshu 心俞), BL-18 (Ganshu 肝俞), BL-20 (Pishu 脾俞), ST-40 (Fenglong 丰隆), HT-7 (Shenmen 神门), P-7 (Daling 大陵), REN-17 (Danzhong 膻中), LIV-3 (Taichong 太冲)

(2) Manic mental disorders
DU-14 (Dazhui 大椎), DU-16 (Fengfu 风府), DU-26 (Shuigou 水沟), P-5 (Jianshi 间使), P-8 (Laogong 劳宫), ST-40 (Fenglong 丰隆)

- **Remarks**

Depressive and Manic Mental Disorders corresponds to Bipolar in modern medicine.

- **Ear acupuncture**

Heart, Kidney, Subcortex, Occipital, Forehead, Shenmen, Sympathetic

1-19 Diabetes 糖尿病 Tangniaobing

- **Differentiation**

(1) Upper Diabetes
Thirst, dry mouth, profuse urination, polydipsia, red tip of the tongue, thin yellow tongue coating, full rapid pulse.

(2) Middle Diabetes
Polyphagia, easy hunger, restlessness, profuse sweating, emaciation, profuse drinking of water, polyuria, dry yellow tongue coating, slippery rapid pulse.

(3) Lower Diabetes
Profuse and frequent urination, turbid urine with sweet taste, thirst and polydipsia, dizziness, blurred vision, red cheeks, soreness and weakness of the knee, red tongue, thin and rapid pulse.

- **Treatment**

  Prescription
  (1) Upper Diabetes
  HT-8 (Shaofu 少府), LU-9 (Taiyuan 太渊), BL-13
  (Feishu 肺俞), BL-15 (Xinshu 心俞)

  (2) Middle Diabetes
  BL-20 (Pishu 脾俞), BL-21 (Weishu 胃俞), ST-44
  (Neiting 内庭), SP-6 (Sanyinjiao 三阴交)

  (3) Lower Diabetes
  BL-18 (Ganshu 肝俞), KI-3 (Taixi 太溪), LIV-3
  (Taichong 太冲), BL-23 (Shenshu 肾俞)

- **Remarks**

  Diabetes is characterized by polydipsia,
  polyphagia, polyuria, emaciation and sweet
  urine.
  Ear acupuncture:
  Pancreas and Gallbladder, Endocrine,
  Stomach, Spleen, Kidney, Lung, Sanjiao,
  Shenmen, Mouth, Center of superior concha,
  Ear apex, Root of ear vagus

1-20 Edema 水肿 Shuizhong

• Differentiation

(1) Yang Edema

It characterized by acute in nature, and firstly show puffiness of the face, eyelids, limbs. The skin is lustrous.

It accompanies cough, asthma, fever, thirst, scanty urine, and lower back pain, superficial rapid pulse.

(2) Yin Edema

It characterized by a slow onset, swelling face is the first stage, and then spreads to the abdomen and whole body.

When pressing on hand, appear rebound slowly. Symptoms are short urine, loose stools, lassitude, weak limbs, pale tongue with white coating, deep thready slow pulse.

• Treatment

Prescription
(1) Yang Edema

BL-13 (Feishu 肺俞), BL-22 (Sanjiaoshu 三焦俞), LI-6 (Pianli 偏历), LI-4 (Hegu 合谷), SJ-5 (Waiguan 外关), SP-9 (Yinlingquan 阴陵泉)

(2) Yin Edema
BL-20 (Pishu 脾俞), BL-23 (Shenshu 肾俞), ST-36 (Zusanli 足三里), REN-9 (Shuifen 水分), REN-6 (Qihai 气海), KI-3 (Taixi 太溪)

- **Remarks**

  Edema refers to retention of fluid in the body and shows puffiness of the head, face, eyelids, limbs, whole body.

- **Ear acupuncture**

  Liver, Lung, Kidney, Spleen, Subcortex, Urinarybladder

1-21 Epigastric Pain 上腹痛 Shangfutong

- **Differentiation**

1. Attack on stomach by Liver Qi
(1) Qi Stagnation
   Epigastric pain, distending pain in the hypochondriac region, nausea, deep and wiry pulse, thin white tongue coating.

(2) Stagnant Heat
   Sudden onset of epigastric pain, restlessness, irritability, dry mouth, discomfort sensation of stomach, red and yellow coating tongue, rapid thready pulse.

(3) Blood Stasis
   Pain, aggravated by food and pressing, vomiting, dark purplish tongue, uneven pulse.

2. Retention of Food
   Distention and pain in the epigastric region, belching, acid regurgitation, pain aggravated after food intake, thick greasy tongue coating, deep slippery pulse.

3. Deficient Cold in the Spleen and Stomach
   The manifestations are dull pain in the epigastric area, and relieved by warmth and

pressing, listlessness, cold limbs, loose stools, pale tongue, weak pulse.

- **Treatment**

Prescription

1. Attack on stomach by Liver Qi

(1) Qi Stagnation

LIV-14 (Qimen 期门), ST-36 (Zusanli 足三里), REN-12 (Zhongwan 中脘), P-6 (Neiguan 内关), LIV-3 (Taichong 太冲)

(2) Stagnant Heat

REN-12 (Zhongwan 中脘), ST-36 (Zusanli 足三里), P-6 (Neiguan 内关), LIV-2 (Xingjian 行间), KI-3 (Taixi 太溪)

(3) Blood Stasis

REN-12 (Zhongwan 中脘), P-6 (Neiguan 内关), BL-17 (Geshu 膈俞), SP-4 (Gongsun 公孙), SP-10 (Xuehai 血海)

2. Retention of Food

ST-25 (Tianshu 天枢), ST-21 (Liangmen 梁门), ST-36 (Zusanli 足三里), REN-12 (Zhongwan 中脘)

3. Deficient Cold in the Spleen and Stomach
BL-20 (Pishu 脾俞), BL-21 (Weishu 胃俞), ST-36 (Zusanli 足三里), REN-12 (Zhongwan 中脘), LIV-13 (Zhangmen 章门)

- **Remarks**

  It may sometimes be caused by emotional disturbance

- **Ear acupuncture**

  Stomach, Spleen, Liver, Sympathetic, Subcortex, Endocrine, Shenmen

1-22 Epilepsy 癫痫

- **Differentiation**

1. During
Experiences headache, dizziness in the chest, followed by unconsciousness, pallor

complexion, clenched jaws, the eyes staring upward, mouthful forms, sleep with big noise. In short time, patients become normal situation, white greasy tongue, thready slippery pulse.

2. After
Palpitation, Dizziness, listlessness, profuse sputum, lumbar soreness, knee weakness, pale white greasy tongue, thin slippery pulse.

- **Treatment**

Priscription
1. During
REN-15 (Jiuwei 鸠尾), DU-14 (Dazhui 大椎), DU-26 (Shuigou 水沟), P-5 (Jianshi 间使), LIV-3 (Taichong 太冲), ST-40 (Fenglong 丰隆)

2. After
HT-7 (Shenmen 神门), SP-6 (Sanyinjiao 三阴交), KI-3 (Taixi 太溪), BL-15 (Xinshu 心俞), EX-HN3 (Yintang 印堂), EX-B9 (Yaoqi 腰奇)

- **Remarks**

It is characterized a sudden falling down in a fit, mouthful forms, eyes staring upward, with large noise of sleep at the place.

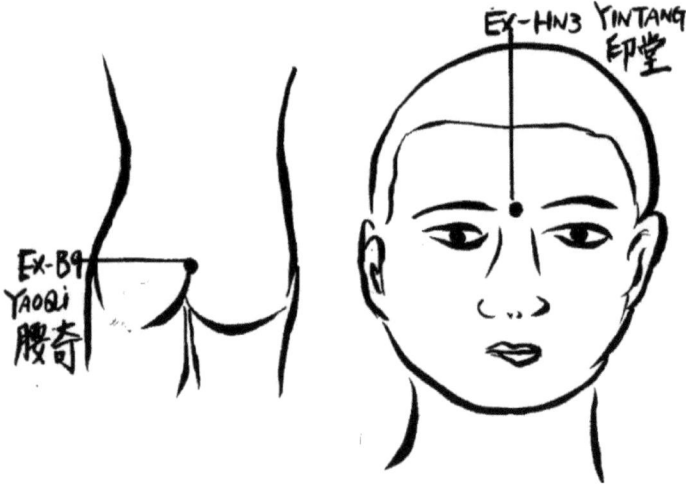

1-23 Facial Pain 面部疼痛 Mianbutengtong

- **Differentiation**

1. Wind-Cold
   Pain cheek, facial spasm aggravation of pain, headache, aversion to cold thin white tongue coating, wiry tense pulse.

2. Wind-Heat
   Burning pain in the cheek, feverish sensation on one side of the face, eye congestion, dry mouth and throat, yellow thin tongue coating, wiry rapid pulse.

3. Liver and Stomach Heat Excess
   Cheek burning pain, restlessness, congestion of the eye, dizziness, fullness of chest, distention in the hypochondriac region, constipation, dry red tongue, thick yellow coating, wiry rapid pulse.

4. Fire Hyperactivity by Yin Deficiency
   Cheek pain, dizziness, blurring of vision, feverish sensation in the palms and soles, red and less coating tongue, thin rapid pulse.

- **Treatment**

  Prescription: Based pm the pain location.
  (1) Forehead pain
     BL-2 (Zanzhu 攒竹), GB-14 (Yangbai 阳白),
     GB-8 (Shuaigu 率谷), ST-8 (Touwei 头维),
     SJ-3 (Zhongzhu 中诸)

  (2) Superior maxillary pain
     ST-2 (Sibai 四白), SI-18 (Quanliao 颧髎), LI-
     20 (Yingxiang 迎香), LI-4 (Hegu 合谷), EX-
     HN5 (Taiyang 太阳)

  (3) Inferior maxillary pain
     REN-24 (Chengjiang 承浆), SJ-17 (Yifeng 翳
     风), ST-6 (Jiache 颊车), ST-7 (Xiaguan 下关)

- **Remarks**

  It mostly affects one side of the face. It is like
  Trigeminal neuralgia in modern medicine.

- **Ear acupuncture**

  Cheek, Forehead, Shenmen, Subcortex,
  Sympathetic

1-24 Frozen Shoulder 肩周炎 Jianzhouyan

- **Differentiation**

  Shoulder pain is named in TCM as frozen shoulder or fifty years old shoulder. The exogenous pathogenic wind, cold and damp overcome patients who are exhausted, overstrained, injured, and while sleeping in the shoulder.

  Pain on shoulders alleviates in the daytime and worsens at night. It may involve back. It may aggravate with cold and alleviate with warmth.

- **Treatment**

  LI-15 (Jianyu 肩髃), LI-11 (Quchi 曲池), LI-14 (Binao 臂臑), LI-4 (Hegu 合谷), SI-9 (Jianzhen 肩贞), SI-3 (Houxi 后溪), SJ-5 (Waiguan 外关)

- **Remarks**

It is characterized by a heavy aching on shoulders, and it mostly appears to the person after fifty years old.

- **Ear acupuncture**

  Shoulder, Shoulder joint Clavicle, Sympathetic, Subcortex

1-25 Hiccup 呃逆 Eni

- **Differentiation**

1. Retention of food and stagnation of Qi
   Epigastric and abdominal distension, sticky, yellow tongue coating, rolling forceful pulse.

2. Attack by pathogenic Cold
   Alleviated by hot drinks, white moist tongue coating, slow pulse.

- **Treatment**

Prescription
BL-17 (Geshu 膈俞), REN-12 (Zhongwan 中脘),
REN-17 (Danzhong 膻中), P-6 (Neiguan 内关),
ST-36 (Zusanli 足三里)

- **Remarks**

It is mostly the result of adverse rise of Stomach Qi which is caused by the injury or blockage of overeating of raw and cold food.

- **Ear acupuncture**

Liver, Stomach, Spleen, Shenmen, Sympathetic, Ear center, Root of ear vagus, esophagus

1-26 Hypochondriac Pain 下软骨痛 Xiaruangutong

- **Differentiation**

(1) Stagnation of QI
Distending pain in hypochondrium, fullness sensation in the chest, irritability, thin white coating, wiry pulse.

(2) Stagnation of Blood
Fixed stabbing pain in the hypochondrium, pain worse by pressing, dark purplish tongue, wiry pulse.

- **Treatment**

Prescription
(1) Stagnation of QI
BL-18 (Ganshu 肝俞), Liv-3 (Taichong 太冲), Liv-14 (Qimen 期门), GB-34 (Yanglingquan 阳陵泉), SJ-6 (Zhigou 支沟)

(2) Stagnation of Blood
BL-17 (Geshu 膈俞), BL-18 (Ganshu 肝俞), SP-6 (Sanyinjiao 三阴交), LIV-3 (Taichong 太冲), SJ-6 (Zhigou 支沟), LIV-14 (Qimen 期门),

- **Remarks**

Hypochondriac pain is caused from melancholy and anger which leads to the failure of Liver and QI.

- **Ear acupuncture**
  Liver, Gallbladder, Chest, Subcortex, shenmen

1-27 Headache 头痛 Toutong

• Differentiation

1. Headache differentiation is according to its locality and channels. Pain at the occipital area and neck relate to Bladder channel. Pain at the forehead and supraorbital region relates to the Stomach channel, Pain at the temporal region of both sides and one side relates to the Gall Bladder channel. Pain at the parietal region relates to the Liver channel.

• Treatment

Prescription

1. Points according to the Headache region

(1) Occipital Headache
GB-20 (Fengchi 凤池), BL-60 (Kunlun 昆仑),
SI-3 (Houxi 后溪)

(2) Frontside Headache
ST-8 (Touwei 头维), EX-HN5 (Yintang 印堂),
LI-4 (Hegu 合谷)

(3) One-side Headache
GB-8 (Shuaigu 率谷), SJ-5 (Waiguan 外关),
EX-HN5 (Taiyang 太阳)

(4) Parietal Headache
DU-20 (Baihui 百会), LIV-3 (Taichong 太冲),
SI-3 (Houxi 后溪)

2. Points according to the symptoms and signs

(1) Hyperactivity of Yang of Liver
LIV-2 (Xingjian 行间), GB-34 (Yanglingquan
阳陵泉)

(2) Qi and Blood Deficiency

ST-36 (Zusanli 足三里), REN-6 (Qihai 气海)

- **Ear acupuncture**
  Shenmen, Forehead, Temple, Occiput, Pancreas and Gallbladder, Subcortex, Sympathesis, Spleen

1-28 Impotence 阳痿 Yangwei

- **Differentiation**

It is characterized by the penis inability and erection. The manifestation shows, dizziness, blurring vision, listlessness, poor sprit, frequent urination, weakness knee and lumbar region, insomnia, palpitation, Heart and Spleen may be involved.

- **Treatment**

Prescription
1. Declining QI

REN-4 (Guanyuan 关元), REN-3 (Zhongji 中极), KI-3 (Taixi 太溪), DU-20 (Baihui 百会), BL-23 (Shenshu 肾俞)

2. Declining Heat and Spleen QI
   BL-15 (Xinshu 心俞), HT-7 (Shenmen 神门), SP-6 (Sanyinjiao 三阴交)

- **Ear acupuncture**
  Internal genitals, Kidney, Liver, endocrine, Testis, Excitation point

1-29 Insomnia 不寐 Bumei

- **Differentiation**

1. Heart and Spleen Deficiency
   Difficulty in falling asleep and disturbed sleep, palpitation, poor memory, poor appetite, loose stool, sallow complexion, thin white tongue coating, thready weak pulse.

2. Heart and Kidney Disharmony

Insomnia accompanied by dizziness, tinnitus, leukorrhagia, feverish sensation in the palms and soles, red tongue with less coating, rapid weak pulse.

3. Liver Fire Disturbance
Manifestations are dizziness, short temper, restlessness, hypochondriac pain, thin yellow tongue, wiry rapid pulse.

4. Stomach Dysfunction
Insomnia accompanied by fullness in the epigastric region, abdominal distension, belching, acid regurgitation, yellow greasy tongue coating, wiry pulse.

- **Treatment**

Prescription
1. Heart and Spleen Deficiency
BL-20 (Pishu 脾俞), BL-15 (Xinshu 心俞), SP-1 (Yinbai 隐白), HT-7 (Shenmen 神门), SP-6 (Sanyinjiao 三阴交)

2. Heart and Kidney Disharmony

BL-15 (Xinshu 心俞), BL-23 (Shenshu 肾俞), KI-3 (Taixi 太溪), HT-7 (Shenmen 神门), KI-6 (Zhaohai 照海)

3. Liver Fire Disturbance
BL-18 (Ganshu 肝俞), LIV-3 (Taichong 太冲), LIV-2 (Xingjian 行间), HT-7 (Shenmen 神门)

4. Stomach Dysfunction
BL-21 (Weishu 胃俞), ST-36 (Zusanli 足三里), REN-12 (Zhongwan 中脘), HT-7 (Senmen 神门)

- **Remarks**

In the mild cases, it may be dream disturbed sleep, in severe cases, there may be no sleep for the whole night.

- **Empirical Acupuncture points**

P-7 (Daling 大陵), HT-7 (Shenmen 神门), REN-17 (Shanzhong 膻中), GB-15 (Toulinqi 头临泣), DU-24 (Shenting 神庭), EX-HN1 (Sishencong 四神聪), KI-3 (Taixi 太溪), ST-36 (Zusanli 足三里),

SP-6 (Sanyingjiao 三阴交), LIV-3 (Taichong 太冲)

- **Ear acupuncture**
  Shenmen, Heart, Sanjiao, Occiput, Insomnia point, Subcortex Anterior ear lobe

1-30 Jaundice 黄疸 Huandan

- **Differentiation**

(1) Yang Type
The Jaundice of Yang type is accompanied with fever, thirst, heavy sensation of the body, abdominal distention, fullness in the chest, nausea, yellow greasy tongue coating, wiry rapid pulse.

(2) Yin Type
The Jaundice of Yin type is accompanied with heavy sensation of the body, and with slow over a long duration, nausea, vomiting, no thirst, tasteless, white greasy tongue coating, deep slow pulse.

- **Treatment**

(1) Yang Type
LIV-3 (Taichong 太冲), GB-34 (Yanglingquan 阳陵泉), BL-18 (Ganshu 肝俞), DU-9 (Zhiyang 至阳), BL-19 (Danshu 胆俞), SI-4 (Wangu 腕骨)

(2) Yin Type
BL-20 (Pishu), SP-6 (Sanyinjiao 三阴交), ST-36 (Zusanli 足三里), REN-12 (Zhongwan 中脘), BL-19 (Danshu 胆俞), DU-9 (Zhiyang 至阳)

- **Remarks**

Jaundice is characterized by yellow colour of sclera, and skin and urine. The bright yellow indicates Yang type and dark yellow indicates Yin type.

- **Ear acupuncture**

Liver, Gall bladder, Stomach, Spleen, Diaphragm, Vegus nerve

1-31 Lower Back Pain 下腰痛 Xiayaotong

- **Differentiation**

1. Cold-Damp
   Low back pain occurs often after invasion in pathogenic wind, cold and damp. The pain is characterized by a rapid onset of aching and soreness, stiffness of muscles, limiting extension and flexion of the back. The pain may lead downward to the buttocks and lower extremities that makes the patient feel difficult to bend forward and backward. Pain becomes worse in cloudy and rainy days. The tongue is white greasy, and the pulse is week, deep and slow.

2. Kidney Deficiency
   Slow onset of hidden pain, in the lumber region in mild pain but protracted, weakness of the lumbar region and knee. Symptoms are intensified after strain and stress, white coating tongue, deep thready pulse.
3. Trauma
   There is a traumatic history by patient. The manifestations are fixed local pain and rigidity,

worsens by pressing and turning of the body, dark purplish tongue, wiry choppy pulse.

- **Treatment**

Prescription
1. Cold-Damp
   BL-23 (Shenshu 肾俞), DU-3 (Yaoyanguan 腰阳关), BL-40 (Weizhong 委中)

2. Kidney Deficiency
   DU-4 (Mingmen 命门), KI-3 (Taixi 太溪), BL-23 (Shenshu 肾俞)
3. Trauma
   BL-17 (Geshu 膈俞), BL-40 (Weizhong 委中), BL-32 (Ciliao 次髎), Ashi points

- **Remarks**

It involves the spine which one side or both sides of the lumbar. It refers to soft tissue injury, muscular rheumatism and lumbar disc degeneration.

1-32 Migrane 偏头痛 Piantoutong

- **Manifestation**

  Blurred vision, irritability, hot temper, red tongue with yellow coating, and string rapid pulse.

- **Differentiation**

(1) Pathogenic Wind Invation
(2) Qi Stagnation due to Liver Yang upsurge
(3) Qi and Blood Deficiency

- **Treatment**

(1) One-side of the face
    GB-8 (Shuaigu 率谷), SJ-5 (Waiguan 外关), EX-HN5 (Taiyang 太阳), ST-8 (Touwei 头维), EX-HN5 (Yintang 印堂), LI-4 (Hegu 合谷), ST-4 (Dicang 地仓)

(2) On Head
    DU-20 (Baihui 百会), LIV-3 (Taichong 太冲), SI-3 (Houxi 后溪), EX-HN1 (Sishencong 四神聪),

GB-20 (Fengchi 凤池), ST-8 (Touwei 头维), BL-7 (Tongtian 通天)

- **Ear acupuncture**

Forehead, Occiput, Brain, Neck, Heart, Liver, Ear apex, Helix 6

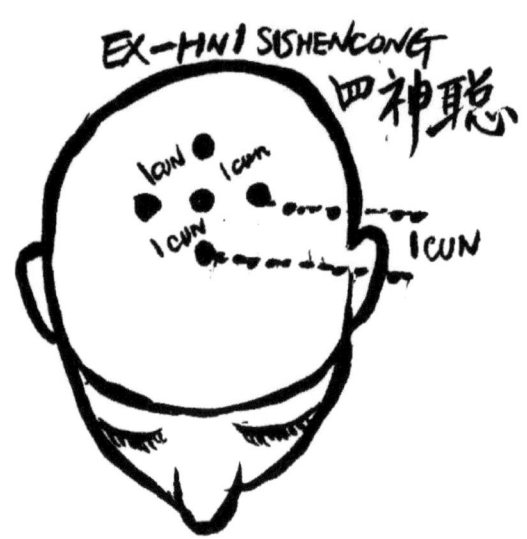

1-33 Nocturnal enuresis 遗尿 Yiniao

- **Differentiation**
  It refers involuntary urination during sleep with dreams at night. It refers involuntary urinary discharge, and it is often seen in children, and it is also mostly seen in the aged patients.

1. Kidney Yang Deficiency
   It happens during sleep, and the patient is not aware of it until waking up. The symptoms accompany with emaciation, lassitude, cold limbs, weak knee and lumber, pale tongue, deep slow pulse.

2. Lung and Spleen Qi Deficiency
   There is frequent and hasty urine, and it accompanies with shortness of breath, lassitude, poor appetite, weakness of the limbs, loose stools, pale tongue slow, deep thready pulse.

3. Damp-Heat
   Frequent urination, occasional enuresis, incontinence of urine, short scanty urine, dripping urine, lower fever, thin greasy tongue.

4. Blood Stasis

The manifestations are abdominal distention, dripping urine, dark purplish tongue, rapid thready pulse.

- **Treatment**

Prescription
1. Kidney Yang Deficiency
BL-28 (Pangguangshu 膀胱), REN-3 (Zhongji 中极), SP-6 (Sanyinjiao 三阴交), KI-3 (Taixi 太溪), BL-23 (Shenshu 肾俞), REN-4 (Guanyuan 关元)

2. Lung and Spleen Deficiency
LU-9 (Taiyuan 太渊), BL-13 (Feishu 肺俞), BL-20 (Pishu 脾俞), SP-6 (Sanyinjiao 三阴交), REN-6 (Qihai 气海), ST-36 (Zusanli 足三里)

3. Damp-Heat
SP-6 (Sanyinjiao 三阴交), SP-9 (Yinlingquan 阴陵泉), REN-3 (Zhongji 中极), BL-28 (Pangguangshu 膀胱俞), BL-39 (Weiyang 委阳)

4. Blood Stasis
SP-6 (Sanyinjiao 三阴交), BL-32 (Ciliao 次髎), REN-3 (Zhongji 中极), BL-17 (Geshu 膈俞), REN-6 (Qihai 气海)

- **Remarks**

  Enuresis and incontinence are related to the function of Lower region, dysfunction of urinary bladder, which the urinary Bladder does not control urination.

- **Ear acupuncture**

  Kidney, Urinary Bladder, Urethra, Subcortex, Lung, Spleen, Sympathetic

1-34 Palpitation 心悸 Xinji

- **Differentiation**

1. Qi and Blood Insufficiency
   The manifestations are lassitude, palpitation, pallor, disturbed sleep, pale tongue, weak thready pulse.

2. Plegm-Fire Disturbance

The manifestations are restlessness, dream-disturbed sleep, irritability, yellow urine, sticky sputum, yellow greasy tongue coating, rapid slippery pulse.

3. Blood Status
   The manifestations are sallow emaciated complexion, palpitation, asthmatic breathing, cold limbs, thready, choppy pulse.

- **Treatment**

   Prescription
1. Qi and Blood Insufficiency
   BL-15 (Xinshu 心俞), HT-7 (Shenmen 神门), P-6 (Neiguan 内关), BL-20 (Pishu 脾俞), REN-6 (Qihai 气海)

2. Plegm and Fire Disturbance
   ST-40 (Fenglong 丰隆), GB-34 (Yanglingquan 阳陵泉), Ht-4 (Lingdao 灵道), BL-13 (Feishu 肺俞), LU-5 (Chize 尺泽), P-4(Ximen 郄门)

3. Blood Status

HT-3 (Shaohai 少海), BL-17 (Geshu 膈俞), REN-6 (Qihai 气海), P-6 (Neiguan 内关), P-3 (Quze 曲泽)

- **Remarks**

  Palpitation is cardiac condition characterized by rapid heartbeat with nervousness and anxiety which may be symptoms in neurosis, functional disorders of nervous system and cardiac arrhythmia.

- **Ear acupuncture**
  Heart, Small intestine, sympathetic, Shenmen, Subcortex

1-35 Poor Memory 记忆力差 Jiyilicha

- **Differentiation**

1. Heart and Spleen Deficiency
   It includes forgetfulness, weakness of limbs, palpitation, poor sleep, pallor complexion, pale

tongue, thin white greasy tongue coating, weak thready pulse.

2. Heart and Kidney Disharmony
   It includes forgetfulness, lumbar soreness, tinnitus, sensation in the palms and soles, restlessness, poor sleep, red tongue, thin rapid pulse.
3. Poor Sprit
   It involves aging. The manifestations ae forgetfulness, poor appetite, lumbar soreness, frequent urination, palpitation, poor sleep, thin white tongue coating, weak thready pulse.

4. Phlegm-Fluid Status
   The manifestations are forgetfulness, low speech, white greasy tongue coating, thin rapid pulse.

• **Treatment**

Prescription
1. Heart and Spleen Deficiency
   REN-6 (Qihai 气海), BL-15 (Xinshu 心俞), BL-17 (Geshu 膈俞), BL-20 (Pishu 脾俞)

2. Heart and Kidney Disharmony

BL-15 (Xinshu 心俞), HT-7 (Shenmen 神门), KI-3 (Taix 太溪 i), BL23 (Shenshu 肾俞), P-8 (Laogong 劳宫)

3. Poor Sprit
   BL-23 (Shenshu 肾俞), KI-3 (Taixi 太溪), BL-15 (Xinshu 心俞), BL-20 (Pishu 脾俞), EX-HN1 (Sishencong 四神聪)

4. Phlegm-Fluid Status
   ST-40 (Fenglong 丰隆), SP-6 (Sanyinjiao 三阴交), ST-36 (Zusanli 足三里), LIV-2 (Xingjian 行间), P-7 (Daling 大陵)

- **Remarks**

  Poor memory is mostly caused by impairment of Heart and Spleen due to overthinking.

- **Ear acupuncture**

  Heart, Kidney, Spleen, Sympathetic, Brainstem, Shenmen

1-36 Retention of Urine 癃闭 Longbi

- **Differentiation**

1. Accumulation of Damp-Heat in the Urinary Bladder
   The manifestations are distention in the lower abdomen, hot scanty urine, thirst but no desire to drink, red tongue with yellow coating, rapid pulse.

2. Kidney-Qi Deficient
   The manifestations are dribbling of urine, lumbar soreness, listlessness, pallor complexion, weakness of knee, pale tongue, deep thready pulse.

3. Urethral Obstruction
   The manifestations are dribbling of urine, pain and distention in lower abdomen, red spot on the tongue, rapid pulse.

- **Treatment**

   Prescription

1. Accumulation of Damp-Heat in the Urinary Bladder

SP-6 (Sanyinjiao 三阴交), SP-9 (Yinlingquan 阴陵泉), REN-3 (Zhongji 中极), BL-28 (Pangguangshu 膀胱俞)

2. Kidney-qi Deficient
BL-23 (Shenshu 肾俞), SP-6 (Sanyinjiao 三阴交), BL-22 (Sanjiaoshu 三焦俞), REN-6 (Qihai 气海), KI-10 (Yingu 阴谷), BL-39 (Weiyang 委阳)

3. Uretharal Obstruction
REN-3 (Zhonji 中极), SP-6 (Sanyinjiao 三阴交), BL-28 (Pangguangshu 膀胱俞), ST-28 (Shuidao 水道), KI-5 (Shuiquan 水泉)

- **Remarks**

The Kidney deficiency causes the dysfunction of the Urinary Bladder which controls urination.

- **Ear acupuncture**

Urinary bladder, Urethra Sanjiao, Kidney, Sympathetic, Subcortex

1-37 Rheumatoid Arthritis 类风湿关节炎 Reifengshiguanjieyan

This is a kind of chronic and immune.

- **Differentiation**

  The manifestations are swelling, stiffness, deformity of the joints, pain. It involves wrist, elbow, knee shoulder, ankle.
  1. Cold-Damp
  2. Damp-Heat

- **Treatment**

  Prescription

  ST-36 (Zusanli 足三里), DU-14 (Dazhui 大椎)

  1. Upper limbs:

     LI-15 (Jianyu 肩髃), LI-10 (Shousanli 手三里), LI-11 (Quchi 曲池), SJ-15 (Waiguan 外关), LI-4 (Hegu 合谷), LI-5 (Yangxi 阳溪), SI-4 (Wangu 腕骨), EX-UE9 (Baxie 八邪)

  2. Lower limbs:

GB-30 (Huantiao 环跳), GB-29 (Juliao 巨髎), EX-LE4 (Xiyan 膝眼), GB-34 (Yanglingquan 阳陵泉), ST-34 (Liangqiu 梁丘), GB-39 (Xuanzhong 悬钟), LIV-8 (Ququan 曲泉), BL-60 (Kunlun 昆仑), ST-41 (Jiexi 解溪), GB-20 (Fengchi 凤池)

(1) Pain:

GB-20 (Fengchi 凤池), SP-10 (Xuehai 血海), BL-17 (Geshu 膈俞)

(2) Limbs heaviness:

LI-4 (Hegu 合谷), LI-11 (Quchi 曲池), SP-9 (Sanyinjiao 三阴交)

- **Remarks**

Moxibution and Ear acupuncture is helpful for curing.

- **Ear acupuncture**

Liver, Spleen, Kidney, Shenmen

- **Empirical acupuncture points**

SI-4 (Wangu 腕骨), LI-4 (Hegu 合谷), ST-44 (Neiting 内庭), SP-6 (Sanyingjiao 三阴交), EX-UE9 (Baxie 八邪)

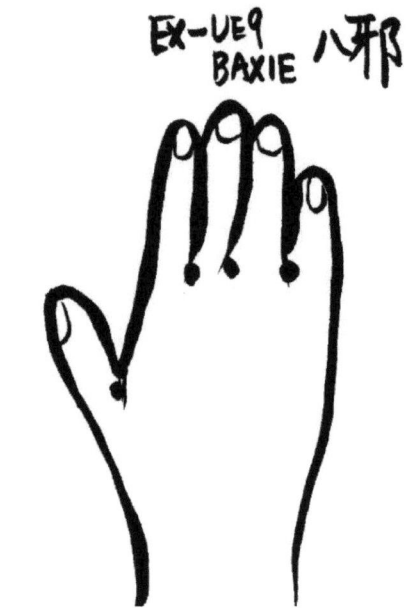

1-38 Seminal Emission 遗精 Yijing

- **Differentiation**

1. Nocturnal Emission
   It may be with dreams,
   dizziness, palpitation, listlessness, lassitude,
   yellow urine, red tongue, thready rapid pulse.

2. Involuntary Emission
   Frequent mission, pallor complexion,
   listlessness, soreness in the lumbar region,
   emaciation, pale tongue, deep thready pulse.

- **Treatment**

1. Nocturnal Emission
   HT-7 (Shenmen 神门), BL-15 (Xinshu 心俞), BL-23 (Shenshu 肾俞), BL-52 (Zhishi 志室), KI-3 (Taixi 太溪), Ren-4 (Guanyuan 关元), P-6 (Neiguan 内关), SP-6 (Sanyinjiao 三阴交)

2. Involuntary Emission
   ST-36 (Zusanli 足三里), BL-23 (Shenshu 肾俞), KI-3 (Taixi 太溪), SP-6 (Sanyinjiao 三阴交), REN-

6 (Qihai 气海), REN-4 (Guanyua 关元), KI-12 (Dahe 大赫)

- **Ear acupuncture**

  Endcrine, Heart, Kidney, Shenmen, Testis, Excitation point

1-39 Shoulder Pain 肩痛 Jiantong

Shoulder pain is named in TCM as frozen shoulder or fifty years old shoulder. The exogenous pathogenic wind, cold and damp overcome patients who are exhausted, overstrained, injured, and while sleeping in the shoulder.

- **Differentiation**

  Pain on shoulders alleviates in the daytime and worsens at night. It may involve back. It may aggravate with cold and alleviate with warmth.

- **Treatment**

- LI-15 (Jianyu 肩髃), LI-11 (Quchi 曲池), LI-14 (Binao 臂臑), LI-4 (Hegu 合谷), SI-9 (Jianzhen 肩贞), SI-3 (Houxi 后溪), SJ-5 (Waiguan 外关)

- **Remarks**

  It is characterized by a heavy aching on shoulders, and it mostly appears to the person after fifty years old.

- **Ear acupuncture**

  Shoulder, Shoulder joint, Clavicle, Sympathetic, Subcortex

  *Refer to Frozen Shoulders.

1-40 Stiff Neck 落枕 Laozhen

- **Differentiation**

It is caused by exogenous pathogenic wind and cold and also while sleeping. Some cases may have the pain spread to the shoulder of the affected side, and it aggravate by movement of the neck.

- **Treatment**
  Prescription
  LI-4 (Hegu 合谷), DU-14 (Dazhui 大椎), Ex-UE24 (Laozhen 落枕), GB-20 (Fengchi 凤池), GB-34 (Yanglingquan 阳陵泉), GB-39 (Xuanzhong 悬中), SI-6 (Yanglao 养老), SI-3 (Houxi 后溪), BL-10 (Tianzhu 天杼)

- **Remarks**

  Combined of GB-39 (Xuanzhong 悬中) and SI-3 (Houxi 后溪), and GB-34 (Yanglingquan 阳陵泉) and SI-6 (Yanglao 养老) make effectiveness on the affected neck. GB-40 (Qiuxu 丘墟). Yuan of GB and neck pain

- **Ear acupuncture**

Shenmen, Neck, Cervical vertebrae, Adrenal gland, Central rim, Occiput, External genital organ

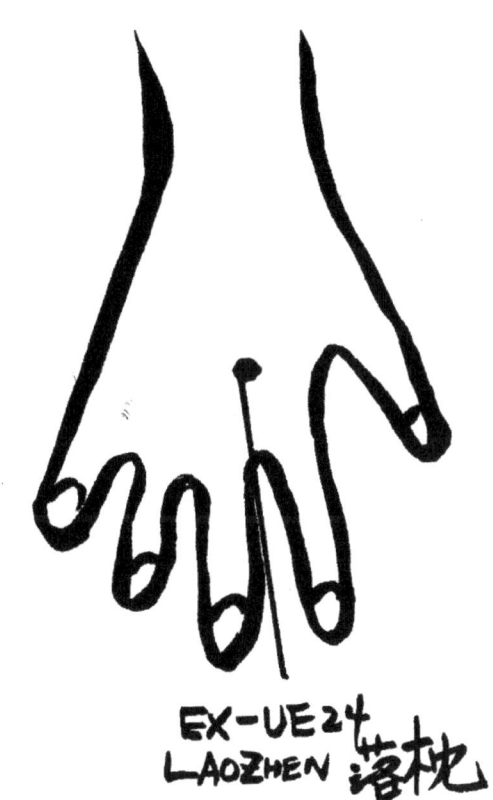

EX-UE24
LAOZHEN 落枕

1-41 Schizophrenia 精神分裂症 Jingshenfenliezheng

- **Differentiation**
1. Heart and Liver Fire Exuberance
   Excitation, mania, not sleep whole night, glowering eyes, increasing the strength, yellow and brown urine, yellow tongue, and rapid pulse.

2. Phlegm and Qi Stagnation
   Mental depression, dull eyes, anorexia, white greasy tongue, slippery pulse.

3. Qi Stagnation and Blood Stasis
   Long-term mania, mental instability, delusion, insomnia, dull complexion, dry skin, purplish tongue, and deep pulse.

4. Heat and Spleen Asthenia
   Depression, palpitation, palpitation, frighten, inactivity, light coloured tongue, and soft and weak pulse.

- **Treatment**

Prescription

DU-20 (Baihui 百会), P-7 (Daling 大陵), ST-40 (Fenglong 丰隆)

DU-26 (Shuigou 水沟), LU-11 (Shaoshang 少商), P-8 (Laogong 劳宫), DU-14 (Dazhui 大椎), SP-1 (Yinbai 隐白), HT-7 (Shenmen 神门), P-5 (Jianshi 间使), REN-17 (Shanzhong 膻中), LI-4 (Hegu 合谷), LI-11 (Quchi 曲池), LIV-3 (Taichong 太冲), BL-15 (Xinshu 心俞), BL-20 (Pishu 脾俞), ST-36 (Zusanli 足三里), SP-6 (Sanyinjiao 三阴交)

- **Electro acupuncture**

  The above prescription points.

1-42 Vomiting 呕吐 Outu

- **Differentiation**

1. Retention of Food

This is characterized by epigastric distention, casting up of sour tastes, belching, abdominal pain, foul gas, constipation, greasy tongue coating, slippery pulse.

2. Invasion of Stomach by Liver Qi
This is characterized by vomiting, acid regurgitation, frequent belching, distention in the hypochondriac region, thin greasy tongue coating, wiry pulse.

3. Weakness of Stomach and Spleen
Sallow complexion, lack of appetite, loose stools, pale, sticky tongue, weak soft pulse.

- **Treatment**

Prescription
1. Retention of Food
ST-36 (Zusanli 足三里), P-6 (Neiguan 内关), REN-12 (Zhongwan 中脘), REN-10 (Xiawan 下脘), REN-21 (Xuanji 璇玑), SP-14 (Fujie 腹結)

2. Invation of Stomach by Liver Qi
ST-36 (Zusanli 足三里), Liv-3 (Taichong 太冲), P-6 (Neiguan 内关), REN-13 (Shangwan 上脘),

ST-21 (Liangmen 梁门), GB-34 (Yanglingquan 阳陵泉)

3. Weakness of Stomach and Spleen
BL-20 (Pishu 脾俞), BL.21 (Weishu 胃俞), ST-36 (Zusanli 足三里), SP-4 (Gongsun 公孙), P-6 (Neiguan 内关), SP-9 (Yinlingquan 阴陵泉)

- **Ear acupuncture**
Stomach, Liver, Sympathetic, Occiput, Subcortex, Shenmen

1-43 Windstroke 中风 Zhongfeng

- **Differentiation**

1. Severe Type Attacking the Zangfu
This condition is critical with sudden onset. The manifestation involves sudden falling down, confused mental state, running saliva from the mouth corner.

(1) Tense Type

The manifestations are sudden collapse, coma locked jaws, clenched fists and jaws, coarse breathing, grey dark tongue coating, wiry rolling pulse.

(2) Flaccid Type
The manifestations are sudden falling down, coma, eyes closed, opening mouth, sweat over head and face, incontinence of urine and stools, flaccid tongue, weak thready pulse.

2. Mild Type (Attacking the Channels and Collaterals)
The condition is mild type. The manifestations are hemiplegia, numbness of skin and limbs, deviation of mouth and eyes, dizziness, yellow greasy tongue coating, wiry slow pulse.

- **Treatment**

Prescription
(Points according to symptoms and signs)
1. Severe Type Attacking the Zangfu

(1) Tense Type
DU-20 (Baihui 百会), KI-1 (Yongquan 涌泉), LIV-3 (Taichong 太冲), ST-40 (Fenglong 丰隆),

P-8 (Laogong 劳宫), DU-26 (Shuigou 水沟, Renzhong 人中),
*12 Jing-Well points of both hands

- Clenched jaws: ST-6 (Jiache 颊车), ST-7 (Xiaguan 下关), LI-4 (Hegu 合谷)

- Gurgling with sputum: ST-40 (Fenglong 丰隆), REN-22 (Tiantu 天突)

- Aphasia and stiffness of tongue: Ren-23 (Lianquan 廉泉), DU-15 (Yamen 亚门), HT-5 (Tongli 通里)

(2) Flaccid Type
REN-6 (Qihai 气海), REN-4 (Guanyuan 关元), ST-36 (Zusanli 足三里), DU-26 (Shuigou 水沟, Renzhong 人中)

- Hemiplegia:
DU-20 (Baihui 百会), DU-16 (Fengfu 风府)

- Upper extremity:
LI-11 (Quchi 曲池), SJ-5 (Waiguan 外关), LI-4 (Hegu 合谷), LI-15 (Jianyu 肩髃),

GB-34 (Yanglingquan 阳梁泉), ST-36 (Zusanli 足三里), ST-41 (Jiexi 解溪)

2. Mild Type (Attacking the channels and Collaterals)

DU-20 (Baihui 百会), DU-16 (Fengfu 风府), ST-9 (Renying 人迎)

- **Remarks**

  It may be applied in Scalp Acupuncture using motor area and speech area.

- **12 Jing-Well points:**
  LU-11 (Shaoshang 少商), SP-1 (Yinbai 隐白), HT-9 (Shaochong 少冲), KI-1 (Yongquan 涌泉), P-9 (Zhongchong 中冲), LIV-1 (Dadun 大敦), LI-1 (Shangyang 商阳), ST-45 (Lidui 历兑), SI-1, (Shaoze 少泽), BL-67 (Zhiyin 至 阴), SJ-1 (Guanchong 关冲), GB-44 (Zuqiaoyin 足窍阴)

- **Scalp acupuncture**
  Motor area, Speech area

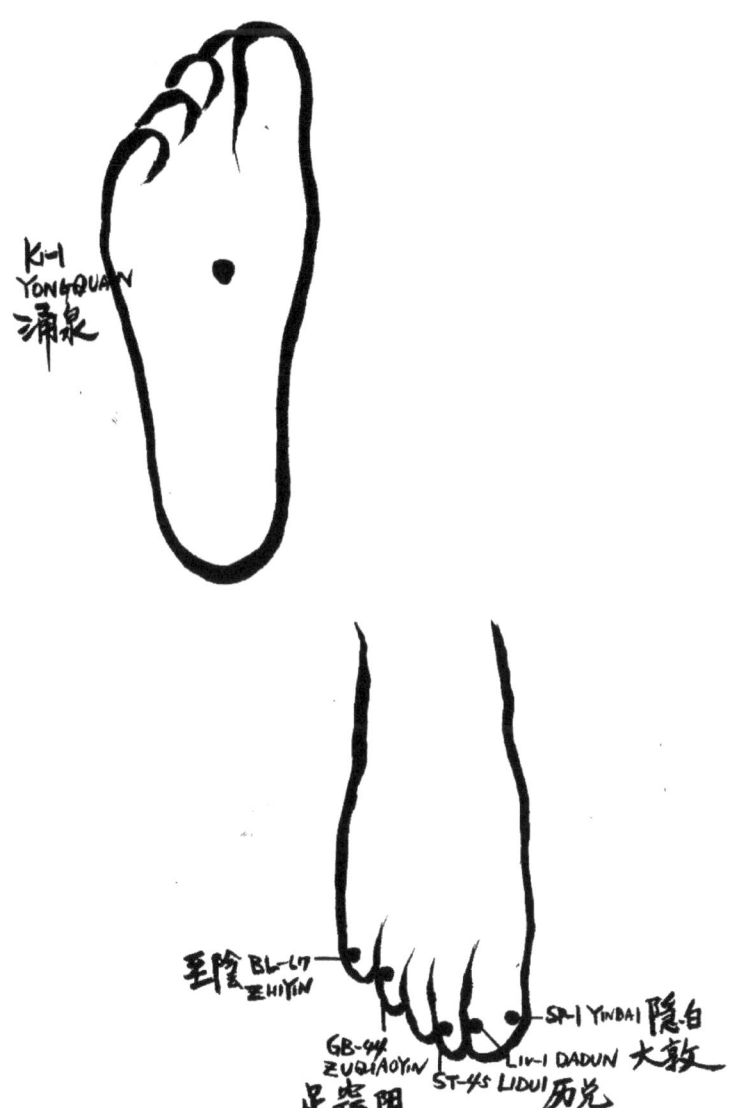

KI-1
YONGQUAN
涌泉

至陰 BL-67
ZHIYIN

GB-44
ZUQIAOYIN
足窍阴

ST-45 LIDUI
厉兑

LIV-1 DADUN
大敦

SP-1 YINBAI
隐白

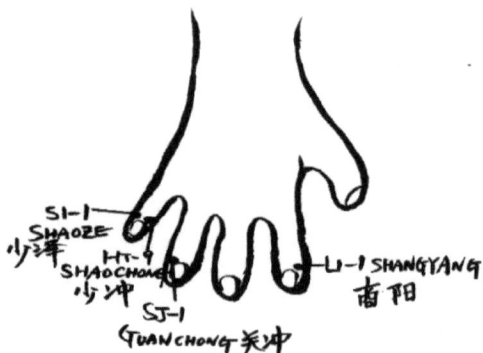

SI-1
SHAOZE 少泽
HT-9 SHAOCHONG 少冲
SJ-1 GUANCHONG 关冲
LI-1 SHANGYANG 商阳

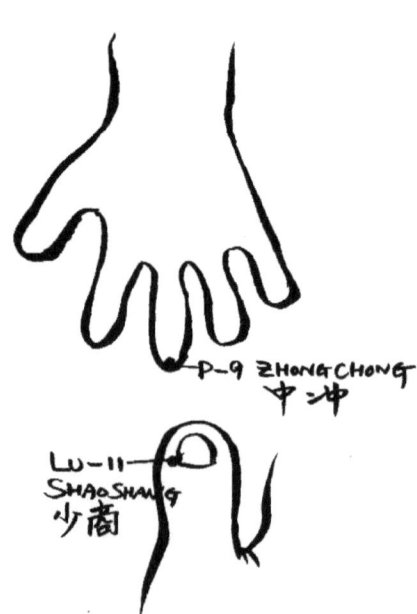

P-9 ZHONGCHONG 中冲
LU-11 SHAOSHANG 少商

1-44 Wei Syndrome 痿症 Weizheng

- **Differentiation**

  Wei syndrome is characterized by muscular flaccidity or atrophy of the extremities with motor impairment.

1. Heat in the Lung
   It usually occurs during or after a febrile disease. Manifestations are fever, cough, restlessness, thirsty, scanty urine, red tongue with yellow coating, thready rapid pulse.

2. Damp-Heat
   The manifestations are heavy sensation of the body, sallow complexion, listlessness, cloudy urine, profuse sweating, hot sensation in the soles of the feet, yellow greasy tongue coating, soft rapid pulse.

3. Liver and Kidney Deficiency
   The manifestations are soreness and weakness of the lumbar region, blurring of vision,

4. Trauma

Contusion causes injury of the meridians and leads to retarded Qi and Blood circulation. As a result, the muscles and tendons are poorly nourished, thin white tongue coating, slow hesitant pulse.

- **Treatment**

  Prescription
  1. Heat in the Lung

- Upper limb:
  LI-15 (Jianyu 肩髃), LI-11 (Quchi 曲池), SJ-5 (Waiguan 外关), LI-4 (Hegu 合谷)

- Lower limb:
  ST-36 (Zusanli 足三里), ST-31 (Biguan 髀关), ST-41 (Jiexi 解溪), GB-30 (Huantiao 环跳), GB-34 (Yanglingquan 阳陵泉) GB-39 (Xuanzhong 悬钟)
  2. Damp-Heat

  BL-20 (Pishu 脾俞), SP-9 (Yinlingquan 阴陵泉)

  3. Liver and Kidney Deficiency

BL-18 (Ganshu 肝俞), BL-23 (Shenshu 肾俞), KI-3 (Taixi 太溪)

4. Trauma
   EX-B2 (Jiaji 夹脊) for spinal injury.

- **Remarks**

  It is seen acute myelitis, progressive myatrophy, myasthenia gravis, periodic paralysis and hysterical paralysis.

- **Plum-blossom needle**

  Points of hand and foot Yangming meridians, EX-B2 (Jiaji 夹脊)

Charpter 2. Gynecology

2-1 Amenorrhea 闭经 Bijing

- **Differentiation**

1. Blood Stasis
   This type of Amenorrhea is characterized by an absence of menses, distention and pain in the lower abdomen, aggravated by pressing, but relieved by warmth, purplish dark tongue, deep wiry pulse.

2. Blood Deficiency
   This type of Amenorrhea is characterized by delayed menstrual period, and gradually decreasing in amount of flow. It is accompanied by soreness in the lumbar region and knees, dizziness, loose stool, palpitation, pale, white coating tongue, thready, weak pulse.

- **Treatment**

  Prescription

1. Blood Stasis

REN-3 (Zhongji 中极), LI-4 (Hegu 合谷), BL-18 (Ganshu 肝俞), BL-19 (Danshu 胆俞), LIV-2 (Xingjian 行间), LIV-3 (Taichong 太冲), SP-6 (Sanyinjiao 三阴交), SP-10 (Xuehai 血海)

2. Blood Deficiency

REN-4 (Guanyuan 关元), REN-6 (Qihai 气海), BL-23 (Shenshu 肾俞), BL-18 (Ganshu 肝俞), BL-20 (Pishu 脾俞), ST-36 (Zusanli 足三里), SP-6 (Sanyinjiao 三阴交)

- **Remarks**

This refers to female who does not have an experience to get menstrual flow at the age of 18, and also female who ceased to have menstrual flow over three months.

- **Ear acupuncture**

Endocrine, Ovary, Uterus, Liver, Kidney, Adrenal gland, Heart

2-2 Breast Abscess 乳房脓肿
Rufangnongzhong

This is acute disorder, and it mostly appeared in lactation period after delivery.

- **Differentiation**

  The manifestations are redness, pain, swelling, and accompanied headache, fever, chills, nausea, difficult lactation when it was the early stage.

- **Treatment**

  Prescription
  ST-36 (Zusanli 足三里), LIV-3 (Taichong 太冲), ST-18 (Rugen 乳根), GB-21 (Jianjing 肩井), REN-17 (Shanzhong 膻中), SI-1 (Shaoze 少泽), LI-4 (Hegu 合谷), SJ-5 (Waiguan 外关), GB-41 (Zulinqi 足临泣)

- **Remarks**

  Acute mastitis in modern medicine.

2-3 Dysmenorrhea 痛经 Tongjing

- **Differentiation**

1. Status of Qi and Blood
   This type is premenstrual cramping pain fixed in the lower abdomen.
   Distending pain of lower abdomen with distention in the breast and the hypochondriac region which appears before or after menstrual flow, accompanied by dripping of scanty dark purplish in colour with clots, dark purplish tongue, wiry pulse.

2. Liver and Kidney Yin Deficiency
   This type of lower abdominal pain at late stage of menstruation or post menstruation, and relieved by pressing during or post the menstrual flow. It is mild pain but persistent pain. The scanty flow and pink in colour, may be accompanied by dizziness, palpitation, soreness in the lumbar region and knees, thin white tongue coating, deep thready pulse.

- **Treatment**

  Prescription

1. Status of Qi and Blood

   SP-10 (Xuehai 血海), LI-4 (Hegu 合谷), SP-6 (Sanyinjiao 三阴交), LIV-3 (Taichong 太冲)

2. Liver and Kidney Yin Deficiency

   REN-4 (Guanyuan 关元), BL-20 (Pishu 脾俞), BL-23 (Senshu 肾俞), ST-36 (Zusanli 足三里), SP-6 (Sanyinjiao 三阴交), BL-18 (Ganshu 肝俞)

- **Remarks**

  It refers to the periodic pain, and in severe case, it may be involved the lower abdomen, affecting the lumbosacral region.

- **Ear acupuncture**

  Endocrine, Uterus, Ovary, Central rim, Kidney, Internal genitals, Sympathesis, Subcortex

2-4 Irregular Menstruation 月经不调 Yuejingbutiao

- **Differentiation**

1. Precede Menstrual Flow
   The flow is advanced at least more than seven days, and it may appear fresh red or purple red colour. The symptoms appear irritability, dry mouth, night sweating, feverish palms and soles, red tongue with less coating, rapid thready pulse.

2. Delayed Menstrual Flow
   This condition may the type of deficiency or excess factors. Deficiency caused by deficiency nutrient blood or Yang Qi. Excess caused by stagnation of Qi and Blood of Chong and Ren Channels, which leads to delayed menstrual flow.

3. Disorder of Menstrual Flow
   This condition is mostly caused by impaired circulation of Qi and Blood due to stagnation of Liver Qi, deficiency of Kidney Qi, and the factors are such as emotional depression,

anger, as a result, it become disorderly menstrual flow.

- **Treatment**

Prescription
1. Precede Menstrual Flow
   REN-6 (Qihai 气海), SP-6 (Sanyinjiao 三阴交), SP-1 (Yinbai 隐白), ST-36 (Zusanli 足三里)

2. Delayed Menstrual Flow
   SP-6 (Sanyinjiao 三阴交), SP-8 (Diji 地机), LI-4 (Hegu 合谷), BL-17 (Geshu 膈俞), REN-4 (Guanyua 关元)

3. Disorder of Menstrual Flow
   LIV-3 (Taichong 太冲), SP-6 (Sanyinjiao 三阴交), BL-18 (Ganshu 肝俞), REN-3 (Zhongji 中极)

- **Remarks**

It refers to cycle, duration, colour, quantity. These are related to environmental change and emotional disturbance.

- **Ear acupuncture**

Endocrine, Kidney, Ovary, Pelvis, Internal genitals, Central rim, Sympathesis

2-5 Infertility 不孕症 Buyunzheng

- **Differentiation**

1. Kidney Deficiency
   It relates to irregular menstruations, and scanty flow of light red colour. The manifestations are tinnitus, dizziness, soreness of lumbar region and knee, pale white tongue coating, and deep thready pulse.

2. Blood Deficiency
   It relates to scanty flow light red colour, and delayed menstruation. The manifestations are emaciation, dizziness, lassitude, pale tongue with little coating, deep thready pulse.

3. Cold in Uterus
   It relates to have normal menstruation, but its cycle is sometimes prolonged with dark clots. The manifestations are cold limbs, pain in the

lower abdomen, profuse urine, pale tongue with white coating, and deep slow pulse.

4. Phlegm-Damp Retention
It relates an obese constitution, prolonged cycle, profuse sticky leukorrhea, dizziness, palpitation, white sticky tongue coating, and soft slippery pulse.

- **Treatment**

Prescription
1. Kidney Deficiency
DU-4 (Mingmen 命门), BL-23 (Shenshu 肾俞), SP-6 (Sanyinjiao 三阴交), KI-3 (Taixi 太溪)

2. Blood Deficiency
SP-6 (Sanyinjiao 三阴交), REN-6 (Qihai 气海), ST-36 (Zusanli 足三里), EX-CA1 (Zigong 子宫)

3. Cold in Uterus
DU-4 (Mingmen 命门), REN-4 (Guanyuan 关元), EX-CA1 (Zigong 子宫), Moxibution

4. Phlegm-Damp Retention

REN-3 (Zhongji 中极), SP-6 (Sanyinjiao 三阴交), SP-8 (Diji 地极), ST-30 (Qichong 气冲), ST-40 (Fenlong 丰隆)

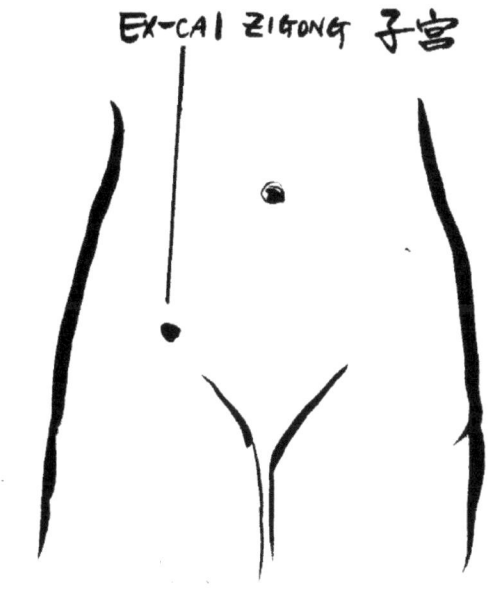

EX-CA1 ZIGONG 子宫

2-6 Lactation Deficiency 乳汁少 Ruzhishao

- **Differentiation**

1. Qi and Blood Deficiency
   It is characterized by scanty or absence of milk after childbirth or decrease in quantity during lactation. The breasts feel soft with no distention. The manifestations are loose stools, lassitude, anorexia, pale tongue with less coating, and weak thready pulse.

2. Liver Qi Stagnation
   There is insufficiency or absence of milk production, and appear anorexia, hypochondriac pain, fullness in chest, emotional depression, irritability, thin yellow tongue, wiry, rapid pulse.

- **Treatment**

Prescription

1. Qi and Blood Deficiency
   ST-18 (Rugen 乳根), SI-1 (Shaoze 少泽), REN-17 (Shanzhong 膻中), BL-20 (Pishu 脾俞, ST-36 (Zusanli 足三里)

2. Liver Qi Stagnation
P-6 (Neiguan 内关), LIV-14 (Qimen 气门), ST-18 (Rugen 乳根), REN-17(Shanzhong 膻中), SI-1 (Shaozeshao 少泽)

- **Remarks**
In TCM, milk is transformed from Qi and Blood.

2-7 Leukorrhea 带下 Daixia

- **Differentiation**
Leukorrhea may be differentiated as white or yellow discharge.

1. Spleen Deficiency
White or slight yellowish of sticky quality without foul smell. The manifestations are loose stool, sallow complexion, lassitude, pale tongue with sticky coating, and slow weak pulse.

2. Kidney Deficiency

It may be much white and dilute quality discharge, accompanied by soreness in the lumbar region, loose stool, frequent urination, pale tongue with white coating, and deep slow pulse.

3. Damp-Heat Retention
It is Yellow discharge with bad odor, and accompanied by itching in the virgina, scanty urination, thirst, sticky yellow tongue, and rapid slippery pulse.

- **Treatment**

Prescription
1. Spleen Deficiency
GB-26 (Daimai 带脉), SP-6 (Sanyinjiao 三阴交), REN-6 (Qihai 气海), BL-30 (Baihuanshu 白环俞)

2. Kidney Deficiency
GB-26 (Daimai 带脉), SP-6 (Sanyinjiao 三阴交), REN-6 (Qihai 气海), REN-4 (Guanyuan 关元), BL-23 (Senshu 肾俞), KI-6 (Zhaohai 照海), ST-36 (Zusanli 足三里)

3. Damp-Heat Retention

GB-26 (Daimai 带脉), SP-6 (Sanyinjiao 三阴交), REN-6 (Qihai 气海), SP-9 (Yinlingquan 阴陵泉), LIV-2 (Xingjian 行间), GB-39 (Xuanzhong 悬钟), BL-32 (Ciliao 次髎), REN-3 (Zhonji 中极)

- **Remarks**

It refers to white discharge of an abnormal colour, quality and odor.

- **Ear acupuncture**

Uterus, Ovary, Endocrine, Spleen, Kidney

2-8 Morning Sickness 孕吐 Yuntu

- **Differentiation**

1. Spleen and Stomach Deficiency
It is characterized by distention in the hypochondriac region with nausea, vomiting ma take place right after food intake or smell of food. The symptoms are accompanied with

dizziness, lassitude, shortness of breath, palpitation, pale tong with white sticky coating, and slow slippery pulse.

2. Liver and Stomach Incoordination
It is characterized by vomiting of bitter or sour fluid. They symptoms are fullness in the chest, pain the hypochondriac region, belching, dizziness, excessive thirst, bitter taste in the mouth, pale tongue, and wiry slippery pulse.

- **Treatment**

Prescription
1. Spleen and Stomach Deficiency
ST-36 (Zusanli 足三里), P-6 (Neiguan 内关), REN-12 (Zhongwan 中脘), SP-4 (Gongsun 公孙) , BL-21 (Weishu 胃俞)

2. Liver and Stomach Incoordination
REN-12 (Zhongwan 中脘), ST-36 (Zusanli 足三里) LIV-3 (Taichong 太冲), P-6 (Neiguan 内关)

- **Remarks**

Morning sickness which is pregnant obstruction, such as vomiting. It is the early reaction of pregnancy during the first three months.

- **Ear acupuncture**

  Shenmen, Kidney, Stomach, Spleen, Occiput, Liver, Subcortex, Pancreas and gallbladder

2-9 Malposition of Fetus 胎位不正 Taiweibuzheng

- **Differentiation**

  Malposition of Fetus means that the fetus is in an abnormal position in the uterus after thirty weeks of pregnancy. It is often seen in multipara or pregnant women who have laxity of the abdominal wall.

- **Treatment**

BL-67 (Zhiyi 至 阴) with Moxibution for 15 minutes for 1-2 times every day until the position of the fetus is normal.

- **Remarks**

Treatment for sitting position on the chair or lies down. According to the history of report shows 80 % of the rate of success.

- **Ear acupuncture**

Kidney, Subcortex, Uterus, Endocrine

2-10 Metrorrhagia 出血性 Chuxiexing

- **Differentiation**
1. Spleen Deficiency
   Sudden profuse metrorrhagia is scanty bleeding in light red colour, lassitude, shortness of breath, poor appetite, loose stool, pale tongue with thin white coating, and weak thready pulse.

2. Kidney Deficiency
   The symptoms include profuse of dripping bleeding of light red colour, cold limbs, soreness in the lower back and knees, pale tongue with white coating, and deep thready pulse.

3. Blood Heat Retention
   The manifestations are deep red colour, restlessness, thirst, constipation, red tongue with yellow greasy coating, and rapid full pulse.

- **Treatment**

  Prescription
  REN-4 (Guanyuan 关元), SP-1 (Yinbai 隐白), SP-6 (Sanyinjiao 三阴交)
- Spleen Deficiency: ST-36 (Zusanli 足三里), BL-20 (Pishu 脾俞)
- Kidney Deficiency: KI-3 (Taixi 太溪)
- Heat in Blood: SP-10 (Xuehai 血海), LIV-2 (Xingjian 行间)

- **Remarks**

Metrorrhagia refers to the uterine type that bleeds irrelevant to the normal menses.

- **Ear acupuncture**

  Uterus, Endocrine, Ovary, Kidney, Spleen, Shenmen, Liver

2-11 Menopause 绝经 Juejing

It is usually seen in woman who is about 55 years old, and at the period before or after termination.

- **Manifestation**

  The manifestations are sudden termination or disorder of menstruation, and flushed face, lassitude, sweating, listlessness, depression, irritability, insomnia, palpitation.

- **Treatment**

ST-36 (Zusanli 足三里), SP-6 (Sanyinjiao 三阴交), LIV-3 (Taichong 太冲), P-6 (Neiguan 内关), HT-5 (Tongli 通里)

- **Empirical points**

Li-4 (Hegu 合谷), LI-11 (Quchi 曲池), DU-24 (Shenting 神庭), SP-6 (Sanyinjiao 三阴交), ST-36 (Zusanli 足三里), KI-6 (Zhaohai 照海), LIV-3 (Taichong 太冲), GB-12 (Wangu 完骨), GB-14 (Yangbai 阳白), BL-2 (Zanzhu 攒竹)

Charpter 3. Surgical and Dermatological Disease

3-1 Acne 痤疮 Cuochuang

- **Differentiation**

  Acne is most cases on face, which may release white bodies upon squeezing. This follows by the formation of small pustules with tidal feverish, itching and pain sensation.

- **Treatment**

  Prescription
  SP-6 (Sanyinjiao 三阴交), LIV-3 (taichong 太冲), LI-4 (Hegu 合谷), LI-11 (Quchi 曲池), GB-20 (Fengchi 凤池), BL-13 (Feishu 肺俞), DU-10 (Lingtai 灵台)

- **Remarks**

  Acne is mostly caused by Heat in the skin such as Wind-Heat and retention of Heat.

- **Ear acupuncture**

Endocrine, Subcortex, Lung, Internal genitals, Ovary, Testis, Adrenal gland

3-2 Eczema 湿疹 Shizhen

- **Differentiation**

1. Acute
   It is characterized by a rapid onset of erythema. The clusters and flakes may break by scratching, and it may turn into severe itching sensation, red tongue with sticky coating, and rapid slippery pulse.

2. Chronic
   After repeated attacking eczema for a long time, it may be caused blood deficiency. The manifestations are roughness of skin, red tongue with less coating, and rapid thready pulse.

- **Treatment**

Prescription

1. Acute
   DU-14 (Dazhui 大椎), LI-11 (Quchi 气海), SP-6 (Sanyinjiao 三阴交), SP-9 (Yinlingquan 阴陵泉), DU-10 (Lingtai 灵台)

2. Chronic
   SP-6 (Sanyinjiao 三阴交), SP-10 (Xuehai 血海), ST-36 (Zusanli 足三里), LIV-3 (Taichong 太冲), BL-17 (Geshu 膈俞), DU-10 (Lingtai 灵台)

- **Ear acupuncture**

  Heart, Lung, Shenmen, Spleen, Adrenal gland

3-3 Goiter 甲状腺肿
Jiazhuangxianzhong/Qiying 气瘿

Goiter is characterized to an enlargement of thyroid gland, causing a swelling in the front part of the neck.

- **Differentiation**

Swelling of the neck, which may be accompanied by stuffiness in the chest, palpitation, shortness of breath, wiry, rolling pulse.

- **Treatment**

Prescription
REN-22 (Tiantu 天突), SJ-17 (Yifeng 翳风), LI-4 (Hegu 合谷), ST-40 (Fenglong 丰隆), ST-36 (Zusanli 足三里), LI-17 (Tianding 天鼎), SI-17 (Tianrong 天容), SJ-13 (Naohui 臑会)

- **Remarks**

It may be caused by anxiety or mental depression which leads to stagnation of Qi and accumulate fluid forming phlegm.

- **Ear acupuncture**

Thyroid gland, Endocrine, Central rim, Sanjiao, Kidney, Liver, Cerebral thalamus

3-4 Herpes Zoster 带状疱疹
Daizhuangpaozhen/Chanyaohuodan

It is known as heat rash and it mostly affects the lumbar region.

- **Differentiation**

  It occurs mainly small vesicles such as beads forming mostly in the lumbar region and the waist with red coloured blisters. The manifestations are burning pain sensation.

- **Treatment**

  Prescription
  LI-11 (Quchi 曲池), SP-10 (Xuehai 血海), BL-40 (Weizhong 委中), EX-B2 (Jiaji 夹脊), GB-34 (Yanglingquan 阳陵泉)

  Addition: according type
  1. Wind-Heat type
  LIV-2 (Xingjian 行间), LIV-3 (Taichong 太冲), GB-44 (Zuqiaoyin 足窍阴), GB-41 (Zulinqi 足临泣), DU-10 (Lingtai 灵台), SJ-6 (Zhigou 支沟)

2. Damp-Heat type
   SP-4 (Gongsun 公孙), SJ-5 (Waiguan 外关), ST-44 (Neiting 内庭), ST-36 (Zusanli 足三里), GB-43 (Xiaxi 侠溪)

- **Ear acupuncture**

  Ear apex, Kidney, Shenmen, Liver, endocrine, Subcortex

3-5 Hernia 疝 Shan

- **Differentiation**

  The manifestations are pain of the testis, lower abdomen, swelling and dragging sensation of the scrotum.
  1. Cold Hernia
  2. Damp-Heat Hernia

- **Treatment**

  Prescription

LIV-3 (Taichong 太冲), REN-3 (Zhongji 中极), REN-4 (Guanyuan 关元), SP-6 (Sanyinjiao 三阴交)

(1) Upper point and Lower point
ST-36 (Zusanli 足三里), LI-11 (Quchi 曲池), SP-12 (Chongmen 冲门), SP-6 (Sanyinjiao 三阴交)

(2) Liver point

REN-6 (Qihai 气海), SP-6 (Sanyinjiao 三阴交), KI-3 (Taixi 太溪), LIV-1 (Dadun 大敦)

(3) Point Zhishanxue (0.5 cun anterior to KI-6 (Zhaohai 照海)

- **Remarks**

Moxibution: point LIV-1 (Dadun 大敦), SJ-4 (Yangchi 阳池), M-CA-23 (Sanjiaojiu)Triangular Moxibution

3-6 Hemorrhoids 痔疮 Zhichuang

It refers to swollen or small pieces of muscle exposed on the anus internally or externally.

- **Differentiation**

1. Internal Hemorrhoids
   Damp-Heat Retention:
   It involves pain in the anus, and small soft swollen veins in fresh red or purplish green colour. The manifestations are feverish sensation in the anus, constipation, red tongue, and rapid pulse.
   Qi Deficiency:
   The manifestation, pallor complexion, shortness of breath, poor appetite, no energy, prolapse of swollen veins, pale tongue, and weak thready pulse.
2. External Hemorrhoids
   The manifestations are visible swollen veins with big size and hard in nature. It may be caused by long sitting, long standing and anus friction which does not involve bleeding.

- **Treatment**

1. Damp-Heat Retention
   LI-4 (Hegu 合谷), LI-11 (Quchi 曲池), LU-6 (Kongzui 孔最), BL-57 (Chengshan 承山), P-4 (Ximen 郄门), EX-UE-2 (Erbai 二白), DU-20 (Baihui 百会), SP-5 (Shangqiu 商丘)

2. Qi Deficiency
   LU-6 (Kongzui 孔最), REN-6 (Qihai 气海), DU-20 (Baihui 百会), BL-57 (Chengshan 承山), P-4 (Ximen 郄门), BL-30 (Baihuanshu 白环俞)

- **Remarks**

  Moxibution with point DU-20 (Baihui 白会), REN-6 (Qihai 气海)

- **Ear acupuncture**

  Large intestine, Spleen, Adrenal gland, Subcortex, Rectum

3-7 Heel Pain 脚跟痛 Jiaogentong

- **Differentiation**

  The manifestations are mainly sprain, pain creating on heel contact with the ground and difficult to walk.

- **Treatment**

  Prescription
  ST-7 (Xiaguan 下关), K-3 (Taixi 太溪), Ashi point

- **Remarks**

  Alternative: Roll the tennis ball back and forth with the sole of your foot many times.

3-8 Neck Sprain 颈扭伤 Jingniushang

Neck sprain is characterized by difficult turning the neck.

- **Differentiation**

  The manifestations are, most patients have limited movement and difficulty to turn to other and back side, and it may be radiate towards shoulder and arm, but no swelling and redness on the skin, thin white tongue, and wiry tense pulse.

- **Treatment**

  GB-20 (Fengchi 凤池), DU-14 (Dazhui 大椎), SI-3 (Houxi 后溪), SI-14 (Jianwaishu 肩外俞), BL-10 (Tianzhu 天杼), GB-21 (Jianjing 肩井)

- **Ear acupuncture**

  Neck, Occipiput, Urinary bladder, Subcortex, Shenmen

3-9 Psoriasis 银屑病 Yinxiebing

It refers to a chronic skin condition characterized by repeated scaled dermatosis, and have some dry silver, white scales covered.

- **Differentiation**

1. Damp-Heat with Wind
   The manifestations are, red tongue with yellow greasy tongue coating, and rapid soft pulse.

2. Blood Deficiency with Dry Wind
   The manifestations are, red tongue with white coating, and thready weak pulse.

- **Treatment**

  Prescription
1. Damp-Heat with Wind
   Li-4 (Hegu 合谷), LI-11 (Quchi 曲池), GB-20 (Fengchi 凤池), BL-17 (Geshu 膈俞), SP-9 (Yinlingquan 阴陵泉), SP-3 (Taibai 太白), ST-9 (Renying 人迎)

2. Blood Deficiency with Dry Wind

LI-4 (Hegu 合谷), LI-11 (Quchi 曲池), SP-6 (Sanyinjiao 三阴交), SP-10 (Xuehai 血海), ST-9 (Renying 人迎), ST-36 (Zusanli 足三里)

- **Ear acupuncture**
  Ear apex, Lung, Endocrine, Shenmen, Heart, Occiput, Subcortex, Adrenal gland

3-10 Scrofula 瘰 Luo

This chronic disorder of the lymph node in the neck region and named beads of tuberculosis. It is commonly shown in children.

- **Differentiation**

1. Early stage
   It does not obviously seen signs. There show several pieces with irregular sizes, without pain and no change of the skin colour.

2. Middle stage
   It is increasing size with pain, red cheeks, lassitude, feverish sensation, and tidal fever.

3. Latest stage
It is developed stage, and it may appear purulent substance of dilute quality like bean curd.

- **Treatment**

  Prescription
  LI-11 (Quchi 曲池), LI-14 (Binao 臂臑), LIV-14 (Qimen 期门), P-6 (Neiguan 内关), LIV-2 (Xingjian 行间), SJ-10 (Tianjing 天井), EX-HN15 (Jingbailao 颈白劳), GB-41 (Zulinqi 足临泣), GB-34 (Yinlingquan 阴陵泉)

3-11 Tetanus 破伤风 Poshangfeng

It characterized by stiffness of back, spasm of tendons, muscles, and limbs.

- **Differentiation**

  It may be painful by invasion of exogenous pathogenic wind into channels. The manifestations are poor nourishment of tendons and vessels, spasm, convulsions.

- **Treatment**

Prescription
DU-14 (Dazhui 大椎), DU-8 (Jinsuo 筋缩), DU-16 (Fengfu 风府), DU-26 (Renzhong 人中) (Shuigou 水沟), BL-40 (Weizhong 委中), BL-62 (Shenmai 申脉), LIV-3 (Taichong 太冲), LI-4 (Hegu 合谷)

- **Ear acupuncture**

Liver, Shenmen, Chest

3-12 Tennis Elbow

This sometimes happen when sportsman's play racket with rotation of forearm and flexion of elbow joint.

- **Differentiation**

The Manifestations are exposure to cold and wind attack to forearm, pain of the lateral side of the elbow, and it is more painful to extending or rotating of the elbow.

- **Treatment**

  LI-11 (Quchi 曲池), LI-12 (Zhouliao 肘髎), Ashi point, GB 34 (Yanglingquan 阳陵泉)

3-13 Urticaria 荨麻疹 Xunmazhen

It is abrupt onset with itching flat-topped wheals of various size on the skin. In TCM, it calls Wind Wheal.

- **Differentiation**

  1. Wind Heat
     The manifestations are red rashes, severe itching, rapid pulse.

  2. Wind Damp
     The manifestations are Light red or white rashes superficial and rapid pulse.

3. Accumulation of Heat in the Stomach and Intestine
   The manifestations are, red rashes, abdominal pain, constipation, diarrhea, thin yellow tongue coating, and rapid pulse.

- **Treatment**

  Prescription
  SP-6 (Sanyinjiao 三阴交), SP-10 (Xuehai 血海), LI-11 (Quchi 曲池), LI-4 (Hegu 合谷), ST-36 (Zusanli 足三里), BL-40 (Weizhong 委中), SP-9 (Yinlingquan 阴陵泉)

- **Ear acupuncture**

  Ear apex, Lung, Endocrine, Adrenal gland, Spleen, Liver, Wind stream

3-14 Vitiligo 白癜风 Baidianfeng

It is characterized by cutaneous white colour of patch which has no symptoms.

- **Differentiation**

1. Vitiligo in local
It characterized by groups of irregular sizes of cutaneous leukoplakia, clear, whitened patches, no itching, no pain.

2. Vitiligo in scattered
It may extend to the body, white colour patches.

- **Treatment**

Prescription
LI-4 (Hegu 合谷), LI-11 (Quchi 曲池), SP-6 (Sanyinjiao 三阴交), SP-1 (Yinbai 隐白), LIV-3 (Taichong 太冲), ST-9 (Renying 人迎), BL-17 (Geshu 膈俞), BL-18 (Ganshu 肝俞), GB-20 (Fengchi 凤池)

- **Ear acupuncuture**

Lung, Spleen, Heart, Shenmen, Subcortex, Adrenal gland

Charpter 4. Pediatric Diseases

4-1 Enuresis 遗尿症 Yiniaozheng

It refers to involuntary discharge of the urine of a child. It happens to occur during sleep.

- **Differentiation**

  It may be happened in several nights during sleep. The manifestations are listlessness, poor appetite.

- **Treatment**

  Prescription
  REN-3 (Zhongji 中极), REN-4 (Guanyuan 关元), BL-23 (Shenshu 肾俞), SP-6 (Sanyinjiao 三阴交), ST-36 (Zusanli 足三里)

- **Remarks**

  Moxibution may be applied.
- **Ear acupuncture**

Kidney, Urinary bladder, Spleen, Brain stem, Lung, Subcortex, Urethra

4-2 Infantile Convulsion 小儿惊风 Xiaoerjingfeng

Infants are not physically developed, and they are mentally weak.

- **Differentiation**

1. Acute Convulsion
   The manifestations are high fever, clenched jaws, upward staring eyes, contraction, rattles, rapid and wiry pulse.

2. Chronic Convulsion
   The manifestations are pallor, lassitude, emaciation, intermittent convulsion, loose stools, clear urine, week pulse.

- **Treatment**

Prescription

LI-11 (Quchi 曲池), DU-26 (Renzhong 人中, Shuigou 水沟), EX-UE-11 (Shixuan 十宣)

1. Points for different symptoms and sign

Protracted Convulsion: LIV-2 (Xingjian 行间), GB-34 (Yanglingquan 阳陵泉), BL-60 (Kunlun 昆仑), SI-3 (Houxi 后溪)

High Fever: LI-4 (Hegu 合谷), DU-14 (Dazhui 大椎)

Coma: KI-1 (Yongquan 涌泉), P-8 (Laogong 劳宫)

- **Remarks**

  Point EX-UE-11 (Shixuan 十宣) locates on the tips of the ten fingers, 0.1 cun distal to end of the nails.

- **Ear acupuncture**

  Shenmen, Sympathetic, Brain stem, Subcortex, Heart, Kidney, Stomach, Spleen

4-3 Infantile Diarrhea 小儿腹泻 Xiaoerfuxie

It is a common pediatric disease, mainly manifested by frequent bowel movement, watery feces. It may occur in any season, but more often occurs in summer and autumn.

- **Differentiation**

1. Cold-Damp

   The stool is watery, abdominal pain, accompanied by aversion to cold, pale tongue with thin coating, and thin deep pulse.

2. Damp-Heat
   The manifestations are the yellowish stool, watery, feverish sensation, yellow and greasy tongue coating, slippery rapid pulse.

3. Food Retention
   The manifestations are epigastric distension that alleviated by bowel movement, poor appetite, vomiting, thick yellow greasy tongue coating, full slippery pulse.

4. Yang Deficiency

It characterized by watery stool, cold limbs, poor spirit, pale tongue with white coating, and thready pulse.

- **Treatment**

Prescription
REN-12 (Zhongwan 中脘), ST-25 (Tianshu 天枢), ST-37 (Shangjuxu 上巨虚), EX-UE10 (Sifeng 四缝)

1. Cold-Damp
REN12 (Zhongwan 中脘), ST-36 (Zusanli 足三里), ST-25 (Tianshu 天枢), REN-8 (Shenque 神阙), REN-4 (Guanyuan 关元)

2. Damp-Heat
ST-25 (Tianshu 天枢), REN-12 (Zhongwan 中脘), ST-36 (Zusanli 足三里), ST-44 (Neiting 内庭), LI-11 (Quchi 曲池)

3. Food Retention
REN-12 (Zhongwan 中脘), ST-25 (Tianshu 天枢), ST-36 (Zusanli 足三里), REN-6 (Qihai 气海), ST-44 (Neiting 内庭)

4. Yang Deficiency
DU-20 (Baihuibaihui 百会), ST-36 (Zusanli 足三里), REN-12 (Zhongwan 中脘), BL-20 (Pishu 脾俞), BL-23 (Shenshu 肾俞), LIV-13 (Zhangmen 章门)

- **Remarks**

  The case of catch cold, add point LI-4 (Hegu 合谷).

4-4 Infantile Malnutrition 小儿营养不良 Yingyangbuliang

It is found more often in children under five years old. It is related to the factors of irregular food intake, lactation, parasite diseases, weaken of Qi and Blood, Spleen and Stomach.

- **Differentiation**

  It is characterized by emaciation, listlessness, sallow complexion, loose muscles.

It is accompanied by poor appetite, poor sleep, loose watery stool, pale tongue, and weak thready pulse.

- **Treatment**

Prescription
1. Spleen and Stomach Weakness
ST-36 (Zusanli 足三里), EX-UE10 (Sifeng 四缝), REN-12 (Zhongwan 中脘), BL-20 (Pishu 脾俞), BL-21 (Weishu 胃俞), LIV-13 (Zhangmen 章门),

2. Parasite Infection
ST-36 (Zusanli 足三里), EX、LE (Baicongwo 百虫窝), ST-25 (Tianshu 天枢), REN-12 (Zhongwan 中脘)

- **Alternative Treatment**

Plum-blossom needle
BL-20 (Pishu 脾俞), ST-36 (Zusanl 足三里), BL-21 (Weishu 胃俞), BL-22 (Sanjiaoshu 三焦俞), Ex-B2 (jiaji 夹脊), EX-UE10 (Sifeng 四缝)

4-5 Infantile Paralysis 小儿麻痹 **Xiaoermabi**

It is due to invasion of epidemic pathogenic factors that injure the meridians.

- **Differentiation**

  Paralysis may be the part of body, especially lower limb, and there is muscular atrophy of the affected part with deformity of the trunk.

- **Treatment**

  Prescription
  Upper limb paralysis:
  LI-11 (Quchi 曲池), LI-4 (Hegu 合谷), LI-15 (Jianyu 肩髃), DU-14 (Dazhui 大椎), BL-10 (Tianzhu 天柱), SJ-5 (Waiguan 外关)

  Lower limb paralysis:
  ST-36 (Zusanli 足三里), ST-41 (Jiexi 解溪), GB-30 (Huantiao 环跳), GB-34 (Yanglingquan 阳陵泉), GB-39 (Xuanzhong 悬钟), ST-31 (Biguan 髀关), BL-60 (Kunlun 昆仑), SP-6 (Sanyinjiao 三阴交)

Abdominal muscles paralysis:
ST-25 (Tianshu 天枢), ST-21 (Liangmen 梁门),
REN-4 (Guanyuan 关元), GB-26 (Daimai 带脉)

Hand paralysis:
SI-3 (Houxi 后溪), LI-5 (Yangxi 阳溪), SJ-4
(Yangchi 阳池), SJ-9 (Sidu 四读), HT-3 (Shaohai
少海)

4-6 Mumps 腮腺炎 Saixianyan

This is an acute infectious disease characterized by painful swelling of the parotid region caused by epidemic pathogenic wind.

- **Differentiation**

1. Pathogenic Heat invading the Exterior
   The manifestations are slight fever with aversion to cold, slight yellowish tongue coating, and rapid superficial pulse.

2. Pathogenic Heat Accumulation
The manifestations are pain, feverish sensation, aggravated by pressing, high fever, headache, vomiting, constipation, straw urine, pain and swelling in the testis, red tongue with yellow coating, and rapid superficial pulse.

- **Treatment**

1. Pathogenic Heat invading the Exterior
SJ-17 (Yifeng 翳风), SJ-5 (Waiguan 外关), LI-4 (Hegu 合谷), ST-6 (Jiache 颊车)

2. Pathogenic Heat Accumulation
LI-11 (Quchi 曲池), LI-4 (Hegu 合谷), LU-11 (Shaoshang 少商), SJ-6 (Zhigou 支沟), ST-40 (Fenglong 丰隆), SJ-1 (Guanchong 关冲)
Swelling and pain of testis: LIV-3 (Taichong, 太冲) LIV-8 (Ququan 曲泉)

- **Remarks**
It is also called Epidemic parotitis.

- **Ear acupuncture**
Shenmen, Cheek, Helix 4-6, Ear apex

4-7 Infantile Fever 小儿发热 Xiaoerfare

- **Differentiation**

  It is often caused by attacking of exogenous pathogenic wind, and improper intake of food and milk with retention of food in the interior.
  1. Invading Lung and Stomach
  2. Affecting Blood by Pathogenic Heat

- **Treatment**

  Prescription
  LI-4 (Dazhui 大椎), LI-11 (Quchi 曲池), GB-20 (Fengchi 凤池), SJ-1 (Guanchong 关冲)

  Vomiting and nausea
  Add P-6 (Neiguan 内关)

- **Remarks**
  Add Ear Acupuncture.

- **Ear acupuncture**
  Shenmen, Sympathetic, Long, Ear apex, Trachea, Tonsil, Throat, Spleen, Large intestine

4-8 Whooping Cough 百日咳 Bairike

It is one of the common respiratory infectious diseases, which the seasonal epidemic invasions that produce turbid phlegm in the interior of the body.

- **Differentiation**

1. First stage
   The manifestations are cough, aversion to cold with fever, loss of voice, thin white tongue coating, and superficial pulse.

2. Second stage
   Wheezing sounds in the throat, feels better in the daytime, difficult in the night, straw urine, constipation, yellow tongue coating, and slippery rapid pulse.

3. Recovering stage
   Less cough day by day, spontaneous sweating, hoarseness of voice, red tongue with thin, and thready rapid pulse.

- **Treatment**

  1. First stage
     LU-7 (Lieque 列缺), LI-4 (Hegu 合谷), BL-13 (Feishu 肺俞), BL-12 (Fengmen 风门), DU-14 (Dazhui 大椎), LU-11 (Shaoshang 少商)

  2. Second stage
     DU-14 (Dazhui 大椎), DU-12 (Shenzhu 身柱), ST-40 (Fenglong 丰隆), P-6 (Neiguan 内关), LU-5 (Chize 尺泽), LI-11 (Quchi 曲池), LU-3 (Tianfu 天府), DU-23 (Shangxing 上星)

  3. Recovering stage
     BL-13 (Feishu 肺俞), BL-20 (Pishu 脾俞), ST-36 (Zusanli 足三里), LU-9 (Taiyuan 太渊), LU-7 (Lieque 列缺), KI-6 (Zhaohai 照海), REN-6 (Qihai 气海), ST-25 (Tianshu 天枢), REN-12 (Zhongwan 中脘), REN-4 (Guanyuan 关元)

- **Remarks**

Add Ear acupuncture. Lung, Shenmen, Bronchus, Sympathetic.

- **Ear acupuncture**
  Lung, Shenmen, Sympathetic, Trachea

Charpter 5. Diseases of Eyes, Ears, Nose and Throat

5-1 Cataract 白内障 Baineizhang

This is divided to Congenital and Acquired.

- **Differentiation**

(1) Congenital
(2) Acquired
This is mainly affecting those over 50 years old and is characterized by chronic disorder in both eyes. It causes deficiency Liver, Kidney, Spleen, Stomach, Yin deficiency and is failure the essence and blood to prevent eye malnourishment.

- **Treatment**

Prescription
BL-1 (Jingming 睛明), GB-14 (Yangbai 阳白), GB-20 (Fengchi 凤池), LI-4 (Hegu 合谷), EX-HN7 (Qiuhou 球后), EX-HN5 (Taiyang 太阳), EX-HN14 (Yiming 翳明), LI-14 (Binao 臂臑),

GB-1 (Tongziliao 瞳子髎), SJ-17 (Yifeng 翳风), GB37 (Guangming 光明), ST-36 (Zusanli 足三里), BL-18 (Ganshu 肝俞), BL-23 (Shenshu 肾俞)

- **Remarks**

Ear acupuncture: Eye region, Liver, Kidney, Adrenal Gland, Heart, Sympathetic Nerve

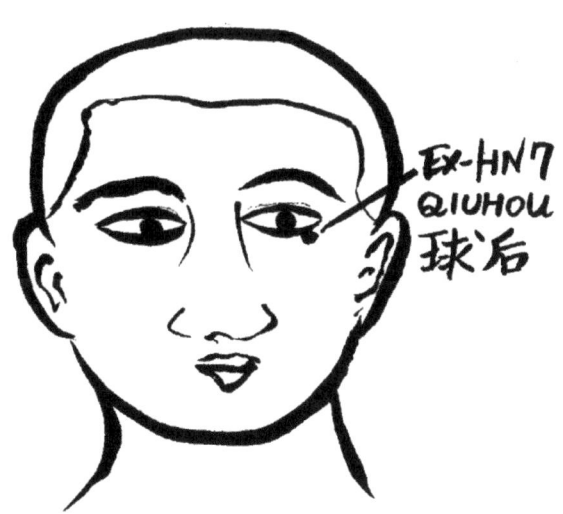

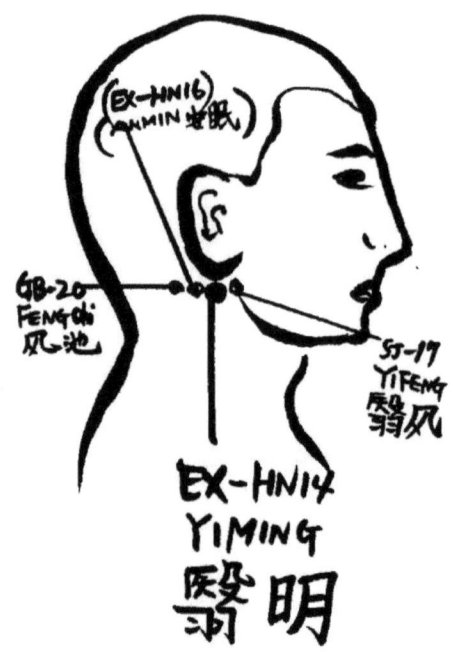

5-2 Conjunctivitis 结膜炎 Jiemoyan

Congestion, swelling and pain of the eye in acute.

- **Differentiation**

Invasion for exogenous wind-heat.
The manifestations are swelling and pain,
burning sensation in the eyelids, and this is
caused by excessive fire in the Liver and
Gallbladder, bitter taste in the mouth,
dizziness, red tongue with yellow coating, and
rapid wiry pulse.

- **Treatment**

  LIV-2 (Xingjian 行间), LI-4 (Hegu 合谷), LI-11
  (Quchi 曲池), EX-HN5 (Taiyang 太阳), DU-23
  (Shangxing 上星), GB-20 (Fengchi 凤池), GB-43
  (Xiaxi 侠溪), LU-11 (Shaoshang 少商), BL-1
  (Jingming 睛明), LIV-3 (Taichong 太冲), GB-37
  (Guangming 关明)

- **Remarks**

  Ear acupuncture: Ear zone

- **Ear acupuncture**

  Ear apex, anterior intertragal, Posterior
  intertragal, Eye, New eye 1-2, Adrenal gland,
  Lung, Liver, Endocrine

5-3 Colour Blindness 色盲 Semang

This is a condition of the person who suffers to identify the brightness and the shape of the objects seen.

- **Differentiation**

  Persons who are unable to differentiate colour upon the objects they have seen.

- **Treatment**

  Prescription
  BL-1 (Jingming 睛明), BL-2 (Zanzhu 攒竹), BL-18 (Ganshu 肝俞), BL-23 (Shenshu 肾俞), GB-20 (Fengchi 凤池), LIV-2 (Xingjian 行间), KI-3 (Taixi 太溪)

- **Remarks**
  Ear acupuncture: Eye zone, Liver, Kidney
- **Ear acupuncture**

  Liver, Kidney, Eye1-2

5-4 Chronic Pharyngolaryngitis 慢性咽喉炎 Manxing yanhou yan

This is caused by recurrence at the acute stage.

Symptoms are, disconfort, itching throat, dryness, hoarseness of voice.

- **Treatment**

  Prescription
  REN-23 (Lianquan 廉泉), LI-11 (Quchi 曲池), LU-5 (Chize 尺泽), LU-9 (Taiyuan 太渊), LI-4 (Hegu 合谷), REN-22 (Tiantu 天突), LU-11 (Shaoshang 少商), P-9 (Zhongchong 中冲), ST-9 (Renying 人迎)

5-5 Dacryorrhea 泪溢 Leiyi

- **Differentiation**

1. Heat tear

It is due to fire and characterized by the running of hot tears against the wind. It caused by accumulation of heat in the Liver and invasion of exogenous pathogenic wind, and it may be exposed Yin deficiency. It is manifested run of hot teas, reddened, swollen eyes, burning pain.

2. Cold tear
The manifestations show lacrimation, thinness of the tears without hot feeling, but it runs of tears to the cheek in some cases.

- **Treatment**

Prescription
BL-1 (Jingming 睛明), BL-2 (Zanzhu/Cuanzhu 攒竹), GB-20 (Fengchi 凤池), LI-4 (Hegu 合谷), BL-18 (Ganshu 肝俞), BL-19 (Danshu 胆俞), BL-23 (Shenshu 肾俞), LIV-3 (Taichong 太冲)

Point for addition of Cold tear:
ST-8 (Touwei 头维), ST-3 (Juliao 巨髎), LU-5 (Chize 尺泽) BL-65 (Shugu 束骨), LIV-8 (Ququan 曲泉)

- **Remarks**
  Ear acupuncture: Eye zone, Liver, Kidney

- **Ear acupuncture**
  Eye, Liver, Kidney

5-6 Deafness and Mute 聋哑 Longya

Deafness is the cause of mute and mute is mostly related to a complete loss of hearing.

- **Differentiation**

  These are referred to complete loss of hearing.

- **Treatment**

  Prescription
  GB-8 (Shuaigu 率谷), GB-5 (Xuanlu 悬颅), GB-9 (Tianchong 天冲), GB-2 (Tinghui 听会), SJ-3 (Zhongzhu 中诸), GB-34 (Yanglingquan 阳陵泉), DU-15 (Yamen 哑门), SI-19 (Tinggong 听宫)

- **Remarks**
  Refer to 5-16 Tinnitus and Deafness.

5-7 Epistaxis 鼻衄 Binü

It refers to nasal bleeding.

- **Differentiation**

1. Lung Heat
   The manifestations are dripping blood by dry nose, dry mouth, fever, cough, red tongue with thin white coating, and rapid superficial pulse.

2. Stomach Heat
   The manifestations are deep red colour, dry throat, constipation, scanty urine, red tongue with yellow coating, and rapid superficial pulse.

3. Liver and Kidney Yin Deficiency
   The manifestations are dry nose, feverish sensation, cough, red tongue with thin white coating, and rapid superficial pulse.

- **Treatment**

   Prescription

1. Lung Heat

LI-4 (Hegu 合谷), LU-11 (Shaoshang 少阳), LI-20 (Yingxiang 迎香), GB-20 (Fengchi 凤池)

2. Stomach Heat
LI-4 (Hegu 合谷), LI-20 (Yingxiang 迎香), DU-23 (Shangxing 上星), ST-45 (Lidui 厉兑), ST-44 (Neiting 内庭)

3. Liver and Kidney Yin Deficiency
KI-3 (Taixi 太溪), LIV-3 (Taichong 太冲), BL-7 (Tongtian 通天), BL-58 (Feiyang 飞扬)

- **Remarks**

Epistaxis refers to nasal bleeding caused by traumatic injuries.

- **Ear acupuncture**

Lung, Shenmen, Adrenal gland, Inner nose

5-8 Glaucoma 青光眼 Qingguangyan

It is caused by an emotion which led to fire in the Liver and Gallbladder flaring up the eyes which the fluid could not work properly.

- **Differentiation**

  The manifestations are headache, distention of the eyes, vomiting, congested conjunctiva, cloudiness, and eventually increased optic atrophy, and blindness.

  1. Primary Glaucoma type
  2. Secondary Glaucoma type

- **Treatment**

  Prescription
  LI-4 (Hegu 合谷), LIV-3 (Taichong 太冲), BL-2 (Zanzhu 攢竹), BL-19 (Danshu 胆俞), BL-17 (Geshu 膈俞), BL-23 (Shenshu 肾俞), GB-20 (Fengchi 凤池), KI-3 (Taixi 太溪), SP-6 (Sanyinjiao 三阴交), BL-18 (Ganshu 肝俞)

- **Remarks**

  Ear acupuncture: Eye zone, Liver, Heart, Ear Apex, Hypertensive Groove.

- **Ear acupuncture**

  Ear apex, Pancreas and gallbladder, Liver, New Eye 1-2, Eye

5-9 Myopia 近视 Jinshi

It is characterized in that the eyes can see near objects but not distant.

- **Differentiation**

  It is clear for near objects but blurred vision for distant which may be accompanied by tinnitus, insomnia, dizziness, pale tongue, and weak thready pulse.

- **Treatment**

  GB1 (Jingming 睛明), ST-1 (Chengqi 承泣), GB-20 (Fengchi 凤池), GB-37 (Guangming 光明), BL-18 (Ganshu 肝俞), BL-23 (Shenshu 肾俞)

- **Remarks**

  Ear Acupuncture: Eye zone plus Liver, Kidney Sympathetic point

5-10 Ottis Media 中耳炎 Zhongeryan

It is characterized by pain in the ear and discharge of purulent substance from the ear.

- **Differentiation**

  1. Pathogenic Wind-Heat Invasion
     The manifestations are fever, headache, and foul smell will flow out from the ear, red tongue with yellow coating, and rapid and wiry pulse.

  2. Retention of Damp
     There is a foul smell flows, dizziness, tinnitus, pale tongue with white coating, and weak, thready pulse.

- **Treatment**

1. Pathogenic Wind-Heat Invasion
   LI-4 (Hegu 合谷), LIV-2 (Xingjian 行间), GB-20 (Fengchi 凤池), GB-12 (Wangu 完骨), SJ-1 (Guanchong 关冲), Ear apex

2. Retention of Damp
   ST-36 (Zusanli 足三里), SP-9 (Yinlingquan 阴陵泉), SJ-17 (Yifeng 翳风), SP-1 (Yinbai 隐白)

- **Remarks**

  Ear acupuncture: Ear apex, Kidney, Occiput, Outer ear

- **Ear acupuncture**

  Posterior intertragal, Ear apex, Kidney, Liver, Spleen, Eye, New eye 1-2

5-11 Optic Atrophy 视神经萎缩 Shishenjingweisuo

This is a chronic eye disorder by gradual degeneration of vision.

- **Differentiation**

1. Liver and Kidney Deficiency
   The manifestations are dizziness, tinnitus, dryness of the eye, blurred vision, lower back pain, red tongue with scanty coating, weak pulse.

2. Qi and Blood Deficiency
   The manifestations are lassitude, loose stools, blurred vision, weakness of breath, pale tongue with thin coating, weak thready pulse.

- **Treatment**

   Prescription
   GB-20 (Fengchi 风池), BL-1 (Jingming 睛明), GB-37 (Guangming 光明), EX、HN7 (Qiuhou 球后)
1. Liver and Kidney Deficiency
   BL-23 (Shenshu 肾俞), BL-18 (Ganshu 肝俞), LIV-3 (Taicong 太冲), KI-3 (Taixi 太溪)

2. Qi and Blood Deficiency
   SP-6 (Sanyinjiao 三阴交), ST-36 (Zusanli 足三
   里), LIV-14 (Qimen 期门), LIV-3 (Taichong 太冲),
   GB-34 (Yanlingquan 阳陵泉)

5-12 Rhinitis 鼻炎 Biyan

This is by nasal obstruction and nasal secretion.

- **Differentiation**

  This is induced by the exogenous Wind-Cold
  or Wind-Heat, improper diet, and the
  manifestations are nasal secretion of thick and
  yellow mucosa.

- **Treatment**

  Li-4 (Hegu 合谷), LI-11 (Quchi 曲池), LI-20
  (Yingxiang 迎香), DU-14 (Dazhui 大椎), DU-23
  (Shangxing 上星), DU-25 (Suliao 素髎), LU-7

((Lieque 列缺), BL-7 (Tongtian 通天), SP-6 (Sanyinjiao 三阴交)

- **Remarks**

  Add Ear acupuncture, Nose region (internal, external) Endocrine, Adrenal, Lung.

- **Ear acupuncture**

  Internal nose, External nose, Endocrine, Adrenal gland, Lung

5-13 Stye 麦粒肿 Mailizhong

It refers to the inflammatory furuncle of the sebaceous gland of the eyelid, and often occurs among young people.

- **Differentiation**

  The manifestations are itching, redness, pain, yellow greasy tongue coating, and soft rapid pulse. It may be caused Damp-Heat from

Spleen and Stomach, and accompanies fever, headache, thin tongue coating, rapid pulse.

- **Treatment**

  Prescription
  LI-4 (Hegu 合谷), LI-11 (Quchi 曲池), EX-HN5 (Taiyang 太阳), LU-5 （Chize 尺泽） , DU-14 (Dazhui 大椎), LIV-2 (Xingjian 行间)

- **Ear acupuncture**

  Liver, Eye, Spleen, Ear apex

5-14 Strabismus 斜视 Xieshi

The movement of the eyeball is unable to recognize with both eyes to see the objects in front directly at the same time.

- **Differentiation**

The manifestations show dizziness, tinnitus, blurred vision, pale tongue, and thready pulse.

- **Treatment**

  LI-4 (Hegu 合谷), ST-36 (Zusanli 足三里), ST-2 (Sibai 四白), GB-20 (Fengchi 凤池), BL-23 (Shenshu 肾俞), BL-18 (Ganshu 肝俞)

- **Remarks**

  Ear acupuncture: Eye region, Liver, Kidney

- **Ear acupuncture**

  Liver, Kidney, New Eye1-2

5-15 Sore Throat 咽喉肿 Yanhouzhongtong

It is similar to tonsillitis.

- **Differentiation**

1. Excess Heat

This is abrupt onset with fever, headache, pain in the throat, constipation, thirst, red tongue with thin yellow coating, superficial rapid pulse.

2. Deficient Heat
Gradual onset without fever, dry throat, feverish sensation in palms and soles, red uncoated tongue, and rapid thready pulse.

- **Treatment**

Prescription
1. Excess Heat
LU-11 (Shaoshang 少商), LI-4 (Hegu 合谷), ST-44 (Neiting 内庭), SI-17 (Tianrong 天容), GB-20 (Fengchi 凤池), LU-7 (Lieque 列缺)

2. Deficient Heat
KI-3 (Taixi 太溪), LU-7 (Lieque 列缺), LU-10 (Yuji 鱼际), KI-6 (Zhaohai 照海)

- **Remarks**

Ear acupuncture: Throat, Lung Tonsil, Helix area 1-6

- **Ear acupuncture**

Lung, Tonsil, Throat, Helix 1-6

5-16 Tinnitus and Deafness 耳鸣 耳聋 Erming Erlong

Tinnitus is characterized by continuous ringing of the ear, and Deafness refers to loss of hearing and low degree of hearing.

- **Differentiation**

1. Excess of Liver and Gallbladder

   Tinnitus: It is continuous ringing in the ear and there is no relieving.
   Deafness: Sudden deafness.
   The manifestations are irritability, heavy sensation of the head, bitter taste in mouth, red tongue with yellow coating rapid wiry pulse.

2. Deficiency of Kidney Essence

Tinnitus: It is intermittent ringing and it becomes aggravated after stress and strain, but it is alleviated by pressure.
Deafness: It is gradually intensified deafness. The manifestations are dizziness, lassitude, low back pain, insomnia, red tongue with little coating, and weak thready pulse.

- **Treatment**

Prescription
1. Excess of Liver and Gallbladder
   SJ-17 (Yifeng 翳风), GB-2 (Tinghui 听会), SJ-3 (Zhongzhu 中诸), SJ-21 (Ermen 耳门), GB-43 (Xiaxi 侠溪), LIV-2 (Xingjian 行间), GB-41 (Zulinqi 足临泣), SJ-5 (Waiguan 外关)

2. Deficiency of Kidney Essence
   BL-23 (Shenshu 肾俞), KI-3 (Taixi 太溪), SJ-17 (Yifeng 翳风), SJ-3 (Zhongzhu 中杼), GB-2 (Tinghui 听会), DU-4 (Mingmen 命门), REN-4 (Guanyuan 关元), SP-6 (Sanyinjiao 三阴交)

- **Remarks**

Scalp acupuncture: Hearing region

- **Ear acupuncture**

Internal ear, Occiput, Pancreas and gallbladder, Kidney, Sympathesis, Root of ear vagus, Adrenal gland

5-17 Toothache 齿痛 Chitong

- **Difference**

  1. Wind-Heat
     Toothache follows swelling, pain, preference for cold food, fever, constipation, red tongue with white coating, and rapid pulse.

  2. Kidney Deficiency
     Toothache follows intermittent pain, loose teeth, red tongue, and rapid thready pulse.

- **Treatment**

Prescription

1. Wind-Heat
   ST-44 (Neiting 内庭), GB-20 (Fengchi 凤池), LI-4 (Hegu 合谷), ST-6 (Jiache 颊车), ST-7 (Xiaguan 下关)

2. Kidney Deficiency
   KI-3 (Taixi 太溪), LI-4 (Hegu 合谷), ST-6 (Jiach 颊车), ST-7 (Xiaguan 下关)

   *Refer to 5-16 Deafness and Mute

- **Ear acupuncture**
  Lower jaw, Upper jaw, Shenmen, Toothache point

5-18 Tonsillitis 扁桃体炎 Biantaotiyan

It is caused by inflammation by the invasion of streptococcus and staphylococcus.

- **Differentiation**

  The symptom is marked by swelling, pain, fever, headache.
  1. Wind-Heat
  2. Deficiency of Kidney Yin

- **Treatment**

  Prescription
  LU-11 (Shaoshang 少商), LI-1 (Shangyang 商阳), LIV-1 (Dadun 大敦), SI-11 (Tianrong 天容), LI-4 (Hegu 合谷), ST-44 (Neiting 内庭), LI-11 (Quchi 曲池), KI-3 (Taixi 太溪), LU-7 (Lieque 列缺), SJ-3 (Zhongzhu 中诸)

5-19 Trigeminal Neuralgia 三叉神经痛 Sanchashenjingtong

Trigeminal nerves are divided into three branches, which are supraorbital branch, maxillary branch and mandibular branch.

- **Differentiation**

It is manifested by sudden onset of facial pain, occurs in transient paroxysms, and just like being cutting, burning and needling, which lasts in a few seconds or few minutes, and several times a day. It is accompanied by local spasm, lacrimation and salivation.

- **Treatment**

Prescription
(1) Main points:
ST-44 (Neiting 内庭), LI-4 (Hegu 合谷), ST-7 (Xiaguan 下关)

(2) Then, combine the other points according to different symptoms and pain location.

ST-2 (Sibai 四白), ST-6 (Jiache 颊车), ST-4 (Dicang 地仓), REN-24 (Chengjian 承浆), GB-14 (Yangbai 阳白), BL-2 (Cuanzhu, zanzhu 攒竹), SJ-3 (Zhongzhu 中诸), GB-41 (Zulinqi 足临泣), LIV-3 (Taichong 太冲), EX-HN5 (Taiyang 太阳), EX-HN4 (Yuyao 鱼腰)

- **Remarks**

  Trigeminal Neuralgia is referred to Facial pain.

- **Ear acupuncture**

  Cheek, Forehead, Shenmen, Subcortex, Sympathetic

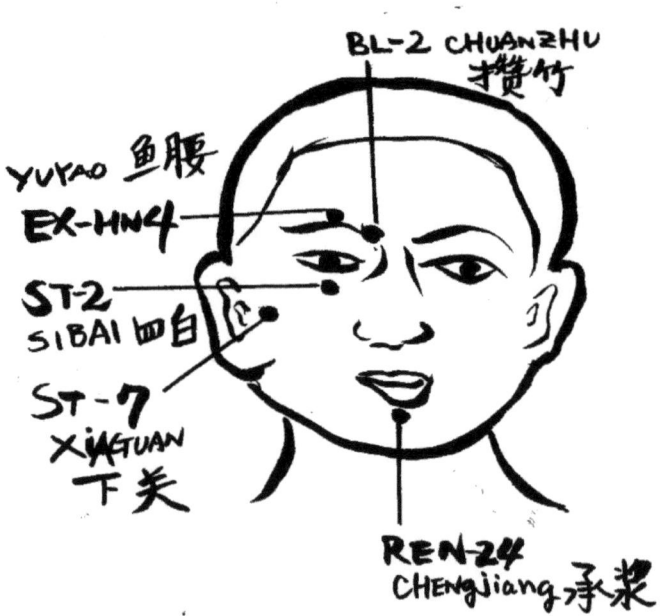

Charpter 6.   Miscellaneous

6-1 Alopecia 脱发症 Tuofazheng

The hair falls off in patches on head where is completely bold.

- **Differentiation**

    It may be caused by mental stress, anxiety, sudden nervous shock.
    (1) Liver and Kidney Yin Deficiency

- **Treatment**

    Plum-blossom needle: tap slight gradually use more quickly and harder a little on the affected area. It becomes congested, red colour, bleeding for about 15 min. after tapping. After that, let to rub the skin on bald area with fresh ginger. It is the best to do 1-2 times a week for some month.

6-2 Cervical Spondylopathy 颈椎病 Jingchuibing

- **Manifestation**

  Pain in the around the neck, forearm, shoulder, movement of the head, numbness in the lower limbs, heavy sensation, dizziness, headache.

- **Treatment**

  Prescription
  GB-20 (Fengchi 凤池), LI-11 (Quchi 曲池), LI-15 (Jianyu 肩髃), LI-4 (Hegu 合谷), SI-3 (Houxi 后溪), EX-B2 (Jiaji 夹脊), ST-36 (Zusanli 足三里), GB-34 (Yanlingquan 阳陵泉)

- **Alternative treatment**

  Plum blossom Needle:
  EX-B2 (Jiaji 夹脊)

6-3 Cosmesis 美容 Meirong

Cosmetic acupuncture, which helps to promote Qi and Blood circulation by needling.

- **Treatment**

  Prescription
  1. Wrinkle:
     GB-1 (Tongziliao 瞳子髎), EX-HN5 (Taiyang 太阳), GB-14 (Yangbai 阳白), ST-3 (Juliao 巨髎), ST-2 (Sibai 四白), SI-18 (Quanliao 颧髎), LI-20 (Yingxiang 迎香), BL-1 (Jingming 睛明), LIV-5 (Ligou 蠡溝), LIV-3 (Taichong 太冲), SP-9 (Yinlingquan 阴陵泉), BL-18 (Ganshu 肝俞), BL-20 (Pishu 脾俞), ST-36 (Zusanli 足三里), SI-3 (Houxi 后溪), LI-4 (Hegu 合谷), SJ-6 (Waiguan 外关)

- **Remarks**

  Ear acupuncture: Endocrine, Cheek, Adrenal, Lung, Shenmen.
  Face massage may be increased to help Qi and Blood circulation.

- **Ear acupuncture**

Lung, Cheek, Endocrine, Sanjiao, Subcortex, Kidney Spleen

6-4 Facial Spasm 面肌痉挛 Mianjijingluan

This is common in women and refers to spasm on one side of the face.

- **Differentiation**

It may be aggravated by fatigue, mental stress, and physical movement.

- **Treatment**

Prescription
LI-4 (Hegu 合谷), ST-4 (Dicang 地苍), ST-7 (Xiaguan 下关), LIV-3 (Taichong 太冲), ST-2 (Sibai 四白), EX-HN5 (Taiyang 太阳), LI-20 (Yingxiang 迎香)

- **Ear acupuncture**

Shenmen, Mouth, Eye, Cheek, Liver, Spleen, Temple, Occiput, Subcortex

6-5 Facial Paralysis 面瘫 Miantan

Deviation of Eye and Mouth 口眼歪斜 Kouyanwaixie

Deviated mouth and eyes are the common name. The paralysis appears mostly on one side, mostly among young and middle-aged people.

- **Differentiation**

  This is caused by weakness of the channels, which are attacked by the exogenous pathogenic wind-cold or wind-heat and led to the flaccidness of muscles by Qi stagnation and blood stasis in the channels of face.

- **Treatment**

  Prescription

ST-4 (Dicang 地仓), ST-6 (Jiache 颊车), LIV-3 (Taichong 太冲), LI-4 (Hegu 合谷), EX-HN5 (Taiyang 太阳), GB-14 (Yangbai 阳白), ST-2 (Sibai 四白), ST-7 (Xiaguan 下关), SJ-17 (Yifeng 翳风), SI-18 (Quanliao 颧髎), LI-20 (Yingxiang 迎香)

- **Ear acupuncture**

  Mouth, Liver, Eye, Cheek, Shenmen, Adrenal gland, Spleen, Forehead

6-6 Facial Pain 面部疼痛 Mianbutengtong

This is a kind of severe pain which is like an electric shock, and occurs in one side of the forehead, maxillary, mandibular regions.

- **Differentiation**

  The pain is cutting, burning and intolerable.
  1. Wind-Cold

Manifestations: Abrupt onset of pain, electric shock, pain like cutting, boring and intolerable, several times a day.

2. Liver and Stomach Excess Fire
Manifestations: Pain, irritability, hot temper constipation, yellow dry tongue coating, and rapid pulse.

3. Yin deficiency and Excess Fire
Manifestations: soreness in the lumbar region, lassitude, emaciation, red tongue, and rapid, thready pulse.

- **Treatment**

Prescription
(1)   Main points:
ST-44 (Neiting 内庭), LI-4 (Hegu 合谷), ST-7 (Xiaguan 下关)

(2)   Then, combine the other points according to different symptoms and pain location.
ST-2 (Sibai 四白), ST-6 (Jiache 颊车), ST-4 (Dicang 地仓), REN-24 (Chengjian 承浆), GB-14 (Yangbai 阳白), BL-2 (Cuanzhu, zanzhu 攒竹), SJ-3 (Zhongzhu 中诸), GB-41 (Zulinqi 足临泣),

LIV-3 (Taichong 太冲), EX-HN5 (Taiyang 太阳), EX-HN4 (Yuyao 鱼腰)

- **Remarks**

Facial pain is referred to 5-18 Trigeminal Neuralgia.

- **Ear acupuncture**

Cheek, Forehead, Shenmen, Subcortex, Sympathetic

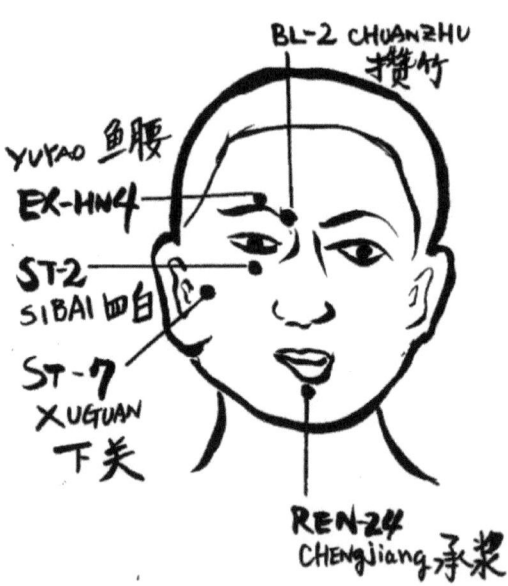

6-7 Goiter 气瘿 Qiying

It is an enlargement of the thyroid gland.

- **Differentiation**

  Swelling of the neck, and accompanied by stuffiness in the chest, palpitation, shortness of breath, wiry and rolling pulse.

- **Treatment**

  Prescription
  LI-4 (Hegu 合谷), ST-40 (Fenglong 丰隆), SJ-17 (Yifeng 翳风), REN-22 (Tiantu 天突)

  Add the point according the symptom:

(1) LIV-QI stagnation:
    REN-17 (Shanzhong 膻中), LIV-3 (Taichong 太冲)

(2) Palpitation:
    P-6 (Neiguan 内关), HT-7 (Shenmen 神门)

(3) Exophthalmos:

SJ-23 (Sizhukong 丝竹空), BL-2 (Zanzhu 攒竹), BL-1 (Jingming 睛明), GB-20 (Fengchi 凤池), EX-HN9 (Taiyang 太阳)

- **Remarks**
  Goiter is described as hyperthyroidism.

- **Ear acupuncture**
  Thyroid gland, Endocrine, Central rim, Sanjiao, Kidney, Liver, Cerebral thalamus

6-8 Hyperthyroidism 甲亢 Jiakang

It is one of the common endocrinal diseases due to excessive secretion of the thyroid gland.

- **Manifestations**

  The symptoms are mental stress, irritability, insomnia, aversion to heat, sweating, low fever.

- **Treatment**

Prescription
LI-4 (Hegu 合谷), SP-6 (Sanyinjiao 三阴交), LIV-3 (Taichong 太冲), ST-9 (Renying 人迎), P-5 (Jianshi 间使), KI-7 (Fuliu 复瘤), HT-6 (Yinxi 阴郄), HT-5 (Tongli 通里), EX-HN16 (Anmian 安眠), HT-7 (Shenmen 神门)

- **Remarks**

- **Ear acupuncture**

  Shenmen, Subcortex, endocrine, Thyroid gland, Heart Lung Dingchuan

6-9 Hysteria 脏躁 Zangzao

- **Differentiation**

1. Liver Qi Stagnation
This type is characterized by restlessness, mental depression, poor self-control, irritability, red tongue coating, wiry pulse.

2. Emotional Depression
This type is characterized by low spirit,
emotional unrest, constant cries with grief or
sorrow, pale tongue with white coating,
thready pulse.

- **Treatment**

Prescription
1. Liver Qi Stagnation
   HT-7 (Shenmen 神门), DU-26 (Shuigou 水沟
   Renzhong 人中), ST-40 (Fenglong 丰隆), P-5
   (Jianshi 间使), LIV-3 (Taichong 太冲)

2. Emotional Depression
   P-7 (Daling 大陵), HT-7 (Shenmen 神门), LIV-3
   (Taichong 太冲), LI-4 (Hegu 合谷), SP-6
   (Sanyinjiao 三阴交), REN-13 (Shangwan 上脘)

- **Remarks**

The causative factor is related to emotional
disturbances such as depression, excessive
joy, anger and grief.

6-10 Obesity 肥胖 Feipang

It refers to excessive accumulation of fat in the body tissues. Clinically, it is divided into Simple and Secondary types.

Simple Obesity: It is due to overeating of greasy, sweet food that exceeds the normal consumption of body heat.

Secondary Obesity: It is caused by hypothalamic pituitary lesions and over-secretion of hydrocortisone.

- **Manifestations**

  Patients have visible fat accumulations in the neck, lower abdomen and buttock. Mild obese patients do not have signs of symptom, but severe patients have metabolic disturbances of aversion to heat, profuse sweating, fatigue, dizziness, headache, palpitation.

- **Treatment**

ST-25 (Tianshu 天枢), REN-9 (Shuifen 水分), REN-12 (Zhongwan 中脘), REN-6 (Qihai 气海), REN-4 (Guanyuan 关元), ST-28 (Shuidao 水道), SP-14 (Fujie 腹結), SP-15 (Daheng 大横), GB-26 (Daimai 带脉), LI-4 (Hegu 合谷), LI-11 (Quchi 曲池), SJ-6 (Zhigou 支沟), SP-10 (Xuehai 血海), SP-11 (Jimen 箕门), ST-32 (Futu 伏兔), SP-6 (Sanyinjiao 三阴交), ST-36 (Zusanli 足三里), ST-44 (Neiting 内庭)

- **Remarks**

Ear acupuncture can be used at the same time as body acupuncture.

- **Ear acupuncture**

Mouth, Esophagus, Stomach, Duodenum, Hunger point, Endocrine, Central rim, Sympathesis

6-11 Occipital Neuralgia 枕神经痛 Zhenshenjingtong

It refers to pain in the occipital and upper cervical areas.

- **Manifestations**

  Pain, cough, sneezing in the occipital area and upper cervical area by movement of the neck. The pain is aggravated in paroxysmal attacks.

- **Treatment**

  GB-20 (Fengchi 凤池), GB-19 (Naokong 脑控), GB-12 (Wangu 完骨), BL-10 (Tianzhu 天柱), BL-60 (Kunlun 昆仑), SI-3 (Houxi 后溪)

- **Ear acupuncture**
  Occipital Neck, Sub cortex, Shenmen

6-12 Stopping Smoking 戒烟 Jieyan

It means eliminating addiction to smoking cigarettes.

In TCM, smoking affects the function of Lung, Heart, Pericardium, Spleen, Stomach, and leads to disfunction of Pulmonary Qi.

- **Differentiation**

  Symptom: Stopping Smoking may be led to restlessness, discomfort in the throat, yawning, blurred vision, weakness, and inability to work normally.

- **Treatment**

  LI-4 (Hegu 合谷), LU-7 (Lieque 列缺), ST-36 (Zusanli 足三里), LU-6 (Kongzui 孔最), HT-7 (Shenmen 神门), SP-6 (Sanyinjiao 三阴交), ST-6 (Jiache 颊车), GB-20 (Fengchi 凤池), DU-20 (Baihui 百会), EX-HN3 (Yintang 印堂)

- **Ear acupuncture**
  Shenmen, Lung, Stomach, Liver, Subcortex, Adrenal gland, Kidney, Liver, endocrine, Heart

6-13 Sciatica 坐骨神经 Zuogushenjingtong

This is the pain radiating to the sciatic nerve distribution in the hip region, posterior lateral aspect of the leg.

- **Manifestations**

1. Primary Sciatica
   It is characterized by a sudden onset of continuous sharp pain, worsens with cold, alleviates with warmth.

2. Secondary Sciatica
   This is a slow onset of pain which may involve primary lesions, radiating pain due to lumbar disc degeneration. The pain is worse with cough, sneezing.

- **Treatment**

   Prescription
1. Primary Sciatica
   GB-30 (Huantiao 环跳), GB-31 (Fengshi 风市), GB-34 (Yanglingquan 阳陵泉), BL-57 (Chengshan 承山), BL-60 (Kunlun 昆仑)

2. Secondary Sciatica
GB-34 (Yanglingquan 阳陵泉), GB-39 (Xuanzhong 悬钟), BL-25 (Dachangshu 大肠俞), BL-26 (Guanyuanshu 关元俞), BL-54 (Zhibian 秩边), BL-40 (Weizhong 委中), EX-B2 (Huatuojiaji 夹脊) L4 to L5

- **Ear acupuncture**
Sciatic nerve, Shenmen, Kidney, Gluteus, Liver, Occiput, Subcortex, Hip, Lumbosacral, Spleen

6-14 Sunstroke 中暑 Zhongshu

It is due to strong sunlight or staying in high temperature time. It mostly happens among elderly and weak people.

- **Differentiation**

1. Mild type
The main manifestations are headache, fever, flushed face, nausea, fatigue, irritability, thirst, rapid thready pulse.

2. Severe type
   The main manifestations are headache, high fever, thirst, short breathing, loss of consciousness, sweating, sudden collapse, deep, forceless pulse.

* **Treatment**

1. Mild type
   DU-14 (Dazhui 大椎), LI-4 (Hegu 合谷), LI-11 (Quchi 曲池), BL-40 (Weizhong 委中), ST-36 (Zusanli 足三里), P-6 (Neiguan 内关), ST-43 (Xiangu 陷谷) EX-HN5 (Taiyang 太阳), REN-12 (Zhongwan 中脘)

2. Severe type
   DU-26 (Renzhong 人中 Shuigou 水沟), DU-20 (Baihui 百会), BL-40 (Weizhong 委中), EX-UE1 (Shixuan 十宣), P-3 (Quze 曲泽), GB-34 (Yanglingquan 阳陵泉)

6-15 Sprain 扭挫伤 Niucuoshang

- **Differentiation**

  The manifestations are local soreness, distension, redness, swelling, and the movement is limited.

- **Treatment**

  Prescription
  Ashi points 啊是穴

(1) Neck:
   BL-10 (Tianzhu 天柱), SI-3 (Houxi 后溪)

(2) Shoulder:
   GB-21 (Jianjing 肩井), LI-15 (Jianyu 肩髃)

(3) Elbow:
   LI-11 (Quchi 曲池), LI-4 (Hegu 合谷)

(4) Wrist:
   SJ-4 (Yangchi 阳池), SJ-5 (Waiguan 外关)

(5) Hip:

GB-30 (Huantiao 环跳), GB-34 (Yanglingquan 阳陵泉)

(6) Knee:
ST-35 (Dubi 犊鼻), ST-44 (Neiting 内庭)

(7) Ankle:
ST-41 (Jiexi 解溪), GB-40 (Qiuxu 丘墟), BL-60 (Kunlun 昆仑)

References 参考文献

1. Zheng Qiwei, Qian Chunyi, Clinical wonders of Acupuncture/Moxibution, 2002

2. Wang Lingli, Chinese Acupuncture and Moxibution, 2002

3. Zhang Yujuan, Practical Handbook on Acupuncture and Moxibution, 1989

4. Geng Junying, Su Zhihong, Acupuncture and Moxibustion, 1997

5. Yu Changzheng, therapeutics of Acupuncture and Moxibution, 1990

6. Deng Liangyue, Chinese Acupuncture and Moxibution, 2008

7. Yan Jie, Skills with Illustrations of Chinese Acupuncture and Moxibution, 1991